FOCAL INFECTION

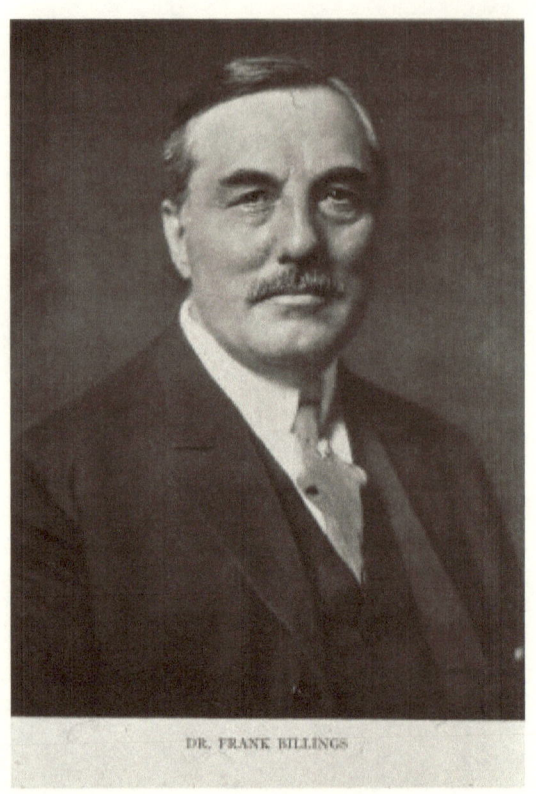

DR. FRANK BILLINGS

"The commonness of infection with the streptococcus, its long story, the widely varying nature of its disease-producing faculties, entitle it to a designation: … chronic streptococcal disease -- the **Billings-Rosenow syndrome**."

Martin H. Fischer
Death & Dentistry, 1940.

FOCAL INFECTION

THE LANE MEDICAL LECTURES

BY

FRANK BILLINGS, Sc.D. (Harv.), M.D.

DELIVERED ON SEPTEMBER 20, 21, 22, 23, AND 24, 1915
STANFORD UNIVERSITY MEDICAL SCHOOL
SAN FRANCISCO, CALIFORNIA

D. APPLETON AND COMPANY
NEW YORK AND LONDON
1916

FOREWORD
S. H. SHAKMAN
InstituteOfScience.com
Santa Monica, Ca. USA
2013

FOREWORD

S. H. Shakman

-- Four Score and Seventeen Years Ago ...

Nearly a century has passed since Frank Billings' 1915 Lane Lecture Series at Stanford University was immortalized in his 1916 book *Focal Infection.* Billings was a big, very big, man. Physically, he was big like a bear according to one colleague. Professionally he was also a giant, having served as President of the A.M.A. in 1902, and he was recognized and revered as a great medical educator. Indeed, Billings is fondly remembered as the father of medical education in America.

Frank Billings had graduated from Northwestern University Medical School in 1881, serving there as professor of medicine through much of the last decade of the 19th Century. Subsequently he was professor of medicine at the University of Chicago for two decades, up until 1924. Beyond his professional responsibilities, Billings was for many years (1906-1912) Chairman of the Illinois State Charities Commission and active in numerous civic affairs, and also served as Chairman of the Red Cross Mission to Russia in 1917.

But it was his work on focal infection that he regarded his greatest accomplishment. Billings had been instrumental in reviving the venerable, sleeping concept of focal infection, the long-recognized notion that infections in the mouth area are related to the cause of diseases elsewhere in the body. In fact, he is generally credited with "coining the phrase". Certainly others had used the term focus or foci in relation to primary infectious sites, but Billings' specific phraseology, in concert with his prominent use of it, and his prominence in general, are to be credited with superseding the term used by William Hunter of England, "oral sepsis".

It was Hunter, in the late 19th century, who was primarily responsible for having kicked off modern-era popularization of the oral focal infection concept; all of the others, including Osler, Mayo, Billings and Rosenow acknowledged this. At the same time it is recognized that Hunter was far from alone in his perspective; for example it is known that Billings himself was actively employing the concept as early as 1886, according to J. S. Marshall of Berkeley, California. (As of that early date, Billings had sent to Marshall several children with enlarged cervical glands, with the request that they be examined for any diseased conditions in the mouth. Marshall had found molars with devitalized pulps and abscesses in all of these patients; all were cured when the teeth were extracted. (*Dent. Summ,*

Jan.,. 1915. p. 14) In any case, it was Billings and his direct legacy that firmly put focal infection on the map and even at the forefront of the medical world.

Of course the relationship between teeth and chronic diseases, particularly arthritis, was known since at least the time of Ashurbanipal of Assyria in the 7th Century B.C. And it was this same circumstance that was to be the cause celebre that would elevate physician Benjamin Rush, a signer of the Declaration of Independence, to the top of his profession in the early 1800s. But although numerous writers through the 19th Century continued to recognize this principle, the development of modern dentistry during the last half of the century tended to obscure it. Then came Hunter's wake-up call.

In the relatively modern times of the early 20th Century, the subsequent work of Billings and his associates – in particular Ludwig Hektoen, Charles Mayo, and the young Edward C. Rosenow -- became widely known. The pendulums of public and professional opinion swung decisively, and properly, to the Billings position. A strong ripple effect of this legacy continued well into the mid-20th Century, as particularly noted in the popularity of tonsillectomy operations through that time. But for the most part, the Billings legacy has been laid aside for the past half-century.

The degree of the demise of this grand legacy in modern times was typified, and perpetuated, in 1976 in the authoritative Bi-Centennial assessment of American medicine, by no less than the acknowledged "doyen" of internal medicine in the U.S., Paul Beeson. Beeson flatly declared that the work of Frank Billings and Edward C. Rosenow was the principal failure in U.S. medicine over the prior century, asserting that it had been refuted by a 1940 article by Reimann and Havens in *JAMA*. Of course one would naturally assume that so prominent a person as Beeson, in so prominent a publication, must have known what he was talking about. A review of the facts indicates clearly that this was not the case.

Beeson apparently had been, indirectly at least, taken in by the same scam that took in all the founders of the modern dental field known as "endodontics", and by association and extension, all of modern dentistry -- a fraud perpetrated in 1928 by an apparently jealous (of Rosenow) bacteriologist, W.L. Holman (*Archives Path & Lab. Med.* **5**, 133), and perpetuated in 1940 by Hobart Reimann (and W.P. Havens, *JAMA*, **114**, 1).

Both Holman and Reimann had previously attempted to discredit Rosenow. As early as 1914, Holman had attempted to discount the facts of Rosenow's remarkable work on transmutations with little more than innuendo, fabrication and arrogant disbelief (*J. Infect. Dis.* **15**:293). Reimann's prominent 1940 attack, beyond its total dependence on Holman for refutation of Rosenow's experiments, was a brief summary of an earlier, 1938 (*Arch. Int. Med.* **62**:305-352) piece by Reimann. That same Reimann 1938 article was, according to Rosenow, "so misleading as to require consideration" in the form of a special and wholly uncharacteristic response (E.C. Rosenow, *Arch. Int. Med.*, **63**, 602-3, 1939.)

In retrospect, it appears that both Holman and Reimann had to be aware that Rosenow's work effectively put them out of business. This was also true for Beeson, although it is not anywhere indicated that either Beeson or Reimann had ever acknowledged, or even recognized, the nature of Holman's deception. Nonetheless, they seem to have been too prepared, even eager, to embrace anything that might be thrown up against Rosenow. They were well aware of Rosenow's thoroughness and the general impregnability of his position, and how it was at variance with theirs. This is also true of the pioneers of endodontics (root-canal "therapy"), but it is nonetheless disconcerting to view the clearly indispensable importance of Holman (and thus the pervasive role of his deceptive action) within the history of dentistry up to the present.

Holman's direct target was a set of data developed by Rosenow, in close association with Billings and others. This data was first presented to the world in Billings's Lane Lecture series in 1915 and subsequently published within this book (see p. 36). This same data was first published directly by Rosenow in *JAMA* in 1915 (LXV, 1688). In summary, Holman's handiwork involved several hundred calculations which converted Rosenow's irrefutable and decisive data into a meaningless and misleading construct. The nature of Holman's deed might be illustrated in the case of stomach ulcers:

Rosenow had found that stomach ulcers with hemorrhages were produced in 60% of 103 animals injected with an organism from patients suffering from this same condition, versus 15% of 405 animals injected with organisms from patients with other diseases. In other words, it was four times as likely that the animals would get the condition if injected with bacteria from patients with it, and it was also noted that the condition was appreciably more severe in the former.

Holman calculated from Rosenow's data that stomach ulcers had developed in a total of 130 animals injected with bacteria from various patients, 62 of which had come from patients with stomach ulcers and 68 of which had come from other patients. He then proceeded to characterize the situation as a 50-50 chance that any localization would occur with one type of bacteria or the other, and falsely asserted that this meant Rosenow's results were inconclusive.

This might all be dismissed as a trivial nitpicking technicality, were it not for the fact that this particular piece of statistical nonsense is at the heart of the foundations of both modern dentistry and modern medicine, to the detriment of the grand legacy of Billings and his school.

It is well now to turn our attention to the grand Frank Billings legacy and his magnificent masterpiece on focal infection. This is the work that Billings himself treasured above all else in his distinguished career -- and he was correct in this assessment. On this foundation and framework constructed by Billings was built a great and solid structure by him and his associates, most prominently Rosenow, one that will surely rule medicine for the next millennium and beyond.

S. H. Shakman
INSTITUTE OF SCIENCE
www.InstituteOfScience.com
Santa Monica, California, U.S.A.
26 January 2013

*Essential technical details of Holman's deceptive action and an overview of Rosenow's work are posted at **InstituteOfScience.com**. For further information, the following related publications by S. H. Shakman are now available *through* **InstituteOfScience.com** and **Amazon.com**

Medicine's Grandest Fraud PhD
Reference Manual Rosenow Et Al. – "Medical Guide of the Future"

INTRODUCTION

The importance of the etiologic relation of Focal Infection to Systemic Diseases has been a subject of study in the clinical material of Rush Medical College, in affiliation with the University of Chicago and the Presbyterian Hospital for the past twelve or more years.

As the study progressed, the attention and cooperation of clinicians and laboratory workers were aroused and developed into a scheme of "team work." This esprit de corps eventually embraced the nursing staff and the patients. Real clinical research was made possible by this cooperative spirit. Living morbid tissues were obtained at surgical operations and also from other patients, who submitted voluntarily and in many instances requested the removal, when necessary under local or general gas anesthesia, of bits of infected tissue (muscle, capsule of joints, lymph nodes, erythematous nodes, fibrous nodes of tendons) of exudates and of the blood, for experimental purposes.

Histologic and bacteriologic studies of this material were made. Animal inoculation was carried on and the lesions of the experimental animals were studied and compared with the morbid human tissues which were the source of the investigation.

Eventually the Memorial Institute for Infectious Diseases, the Otho S. A. Sprague Memorial Institute and the Pathological and Research Department of St. Luke's Free Hospital of Chicago cooperated in the work.

The conclusions based upon the research were not made until a critical survey of the work and the results were investigated by other qualified clinicians, pathologists and research workers.

I may not name, because of want of space, all who have co-operated in the team work, which has made the research a practical success and has opened up a broad field for a more extended study along similar lines. To my clinical colleagues in the college and hospital I extend my grateful thanks. Professors L. Hektoen, E. R. LeCount and H. Gideon Wells have been of invaluable aid to all of us, with advice always helpful though sometimes critical. The members of the house staff have rendered invaluable help by a tireless and enthusiastic bedside and clinical laboratory service. Many of these internes have continued in the work as clinicians, pathologists and clinical bacteriologists. Drs. D. J. Davis, R. T. Woodyatt, H. K. Nicoll, W. E. Post, E. E. Irons, A. M. Moody, F. W. Gaarde, J. J. Moore, and George H. Coleman have done notable work in bacteriology, chemistry, and in experiments upon animals.

The broad significance of the relation of focal infection to systemic disease has been made more definite by the brilliant work of Edward C. Rosenow, who joined the clinic in 1904.

These lectures, therefore, represent the cooperative study of many workers. I have made free use of the results of the labors of all who have aided in the work and I am proud to be their spokesman.

FRANK BILLINGS.

CONTENTS

vii

CONTENTS

LIST OF ILLUSTRATIONS

FOCAL INFECTION

FOCAL INFECTION

LECTURE I

A GENERAL CONSIDERATION OF FOCAL INFECTION

Permit me to express to you my sincere appreciation of the honor conferred upon me, by the Trustees and Faculty of Stanford University Medical School, to give the fifteenth course of the Lane Medical Lectures.

I am complimented also by the fact that the group of workers with whom I am associated, has been engaged in the clinical and laboratory investigation of a subject about which you desire to hear.

Systemic or general disease due to a local infection is a conception as old as medical knowledge.

Long before the development of bacteriology there had been noted many examples of general disease arising from trivial and serious accidental and surgical wounds. The general disease was, as a rule, characterized by chills, fever, and general debility and was often fatal.

The cause was thought to be contamination of the wound or focus with some substance which caused putrefaction. Hence the resulting general disease was called septic. The so-called laudable pus of an uneventful healing wound, when contaminated with putrefactive

1

poison, changed in color, fermented, acquired a bad odor, and, gaining entrance to the blood stream, caused pyemia or septicopyemia. Discussion as to the origin of the putrefactive agents brought forth many theories until the epoch-making discovery of Semmelweis (1847) who traced the constant prevalence of childbed fever in the Vienna lying-in hospital to contamination of the genitalia of the woman in labor by the unclean hands of students and physicians fresh from the dissecting rooms. Cadaveric poison, therefore, was proved to be a cause of childbed sepsis. Local infection followed by embolism, thrombosis and septicemia were recognized as successive stages which were observed in surgical and obstetrical sepsis. E. Klebs was probably the first to recognize that local and general sepsis were due to microörganisms which he termed *microsporon septicum*. But no material gain in practical results occurred until the deductions of Lister, based upon the brilliant researches of Pasteur, that wound infection was due to a *virus animatum* and the rational application by Lister of measures to prevent wound infection. Listerism—antiseptic surgery—was of rapid growth and in its evolutional form as applied today makes general sepsis in surgery and midwifery a criminal offense due to ignorance, carelessness or faulty technic.

But focal infection, which is the subject of these lectures, is broader in its application than is expressed in surgical sepsis.

During the last decade a new interest has been aroused in the subject of focal infection as an etiologic factor of local and of general diseases. The wider discussion of the subject made it appear as a new principle. The wider and broader interest in the subject has been brought about by a better knowledge of bacteriology, of modes of infection, and by cooperative laboratory and clinical research.

A focus of infection may be defined as a circumscribed area of tissue infected with pathogenic microorganisms. Foci of infection may be primary and secondary. Primary foci usually are located in tissues communicating with a mucous or cutaneous surface. Secondary foci are the direct results of infection from other foci through contiguous tissues or at a distance through the blood stream or lymph channels.

SITE OF PRIMARY FOCI

Primary foci of infection may be located anywhere in the body. Infection of the teeth and jaws, with the especial development of pyorrhea dentalis and alveolar abscess, infection of the faucial and nasopharyngeal tonsils and of the mastoid, the maxillary and other accessory sinuses are the most common forms of focal infection. Submucous and subcutaneous abscesses including the finger and toe nails are occasional foci. Chronic infection of the bronchi and bronchiectasis; chronic infection of the gastro-intestinal tract and auxiliary organs of digestion, including cholecystitis, appendicitis, intestinal ulcers and intestinal stasis due to morbid anatomical conditions; chronic infection of the genito-urinary tract, including metritis, salpingitis, vesiculitis seminalis, prostatitis, cystitis and pyelitis, are not uncommon forms. Infected lymph nodes, which are secondary to the primary foci named, become additional depots of local infection. The secondary lymph node infection may persist after the etiologic, distal, primary focus has been removed or has spontaneously disappeared. Other secondary foci may appear in various tissues as a part of the general or local disease which results from a primary focus. As we shall see, systemic and local disease may occur through infection from a focal point by way of the blood stream. This mode of infection is often embolic in character. The tissues so infected may constitute new foci, which in part explains the chronicity of many local and general infections.

ETIOLOGY OF FOCAL INFECTIONS

Focal infection especially of the structures of the mouth and the upper air passages is a very prevalent condition. The incidence of infection of the mouth is enormous everywhere. In addition to the presence of innumerable saprophytes in the mouth and pharynx, one may find in the saliva and pharyngeal mucus, streptococci and staphylococci, micrococcus catarrhalis, pneumococci, diphtheria and pseudodiphtheria bacilli, meningococci, tubercle bacilli and many other pathogenic bacteria. C. C. Bass (1) and others state that endameba buccalis was found in the mouths of 95 and even 100 per cent. of all adults examined. The presence of these infectious microörganisms in the mouth and upper respiratory tract indicates unhealthful surroundings and individual uncleanliness. The individual carrier infects others by contact and by other means.

The character of local infection in various parts of the body is so important that separate consideration must be given to each kind.

Pyorrhea Dentalis and Alveolar Abscess

Pyorrhea dentalis and alveolar abscess (Rigg's disease) is a condition incident to all classes of adults. It is much less prevalent in the young. It is a disease which fundamentally involves the periosteum of the root and neck of the tooth (peridental membrane). It is the chief cause of the loss of the permanent teeth. It may be associated with caries of the crown, and, on the other hand, the crown may remain normal. The infection first attacks the edges of the gum, which may be macerated by decaying food particles between the teeth, or the gum may be injured in masticating hard substances, by toothpicks, and other traumatic agents. Ill health and poor general nutrition make the gums less resistant. The endameba buccalis and various pyogenic bacteria which gain admission to the edges of the gums cause retraction of the soft tissues and the exposed peridental membrane of the neck and root of the tooth become involved in sequence. This periosteum injured or destroyed, there follows softening and ulceration of the soft parts with the end result of acute or chronic alveolar abscess.

Endameba has been known to be a parasite of the mouth for many years. Its relation to pyorrhea alveolaris was first described by F. M. Barrett, (2) in collaboration with Allen J. Smith in 1914. Without a knowledge of the work of Barrett and Smith, C. C.

Bass and F. M. Johns (1) had recognized the relation of the parasite to pyorrhea and had begun experimental treatment with emetin. The endamebas may be found in the gum lesions and they are numerous in the deeper abscesses where they live on the dead tissues. Bass and other investigators believe that the endameba buccalis is the chief etiologic factor in the development of pyorrhea alveolaris.

From the pus and dead material of alveolar abscess and the infected pulp of the teeth, with a proper technic, cultures yield streptococci, chiefly streptococcus viridans and streptococcus hemolyticus, staphylococcus aureus and albus, fusiform bacilli and other less important bacteria. Doubtless the endamebas play an important part in the occurrence of pyorrhea alveolaris and permit infection with the pyogenic bacteria. The bacteria present in the infected areas are the important factors, however, in the causation of general infection from the focus.

Acute and Chronic Tonsillitis and Infection of Lymphoid Tissue in the Nasopharynx

The faucial tonsils are frequently infected through contaminated air, infected food, especially milk, and by direct contact with infected individuals. Many children have large tonsils and overgrowth of other lymphoid structures of the pharynx which make a good soil for bacterial growth. Hypertrophy of the tonsils and adenoid overgrowth in the nasopharynx interfere with respiration, resulting in deformities of the bones of the face and thorax. Obstruction of the upper air passages prevents proper drainage from the nasal cavities and accessory sinuses and leads to infection of the middle ear, the sinuses of the head and the mucous membrane covering the turbinate bodies. In adult life small faucial tonsils may look innocent because of a smooth covering of mucous membrane which seals over infected crypts or an actual abscess. So, too, the stumps of tonsils, the remains of tonsillotomy, may contain infected crypts sealed by the operative scar.

Infected tonsils and adenoids may yield cultures of streptococcus mucosus, streptococcus viridans, streptococcus hemolysans, micrococcus catarrhalis, pneumococci, bacillus mucosus capsulatus, grippe bacillus, diphtheria and pseudodiphtheria bacilli and other pathogenic microörganisms. The tonsils and surrounding lymph tissues may be a focus of tuberculosis from which lymph nodes of the neck and mediastinum may become infected. Smith and Barrett (3) found endameba buccalis in the tonsils of five of seventeen patients. The presence of endamebas in the tonsils would probably favor deep pyogenic infection.

Mastoiditis and Sinusitis of the Maxillary and Other Accessory Sinuses

Mastoiditis as an extension of nasopharyngeal infection through the eustachian tube and middle ear is a serious and frequent disease of the young and occasionally of adults. Members of the streptococcus-pneumococcus group are the usual infectious agents. Staphylococci and influenza bacilli may be the invaders. The proximity of the mastoid cells to the venous sinuses of

the skull makes this focus a frequent source of sinus
thrombosis, bacteriemia and meningitis.

Infection of the accessory sinuses is of frequent occurrence during the changeable seasons. The most frequent bacterial causes are strains of streptococci, pneumococci, micrococcus catarrhalis and influenza bacilli—
less frequently staphylococci. In chronic sinusitis, often
unrecognized, various pyogenic bacteria occur with the
occasional presence of colon bacilli, the bacillus welchii
and various saprophytic organisms. Sinus infection is
frequently chronic because of faulty drainage. When
chronic it may present local symptoms only when a new
"cold" is acquired.

All infectious foci of the head may be associated with
secondary infection of the lymph nodes of the neck and
mediastinum. Kretz (25) records six hundred autopsies with especial reference to the infection of the cervical lymph nodes. In childhood, he says, the superficial nodes of the anterior triangles are involved and soft,
while in adults the deeper glands at the angle of the jaw
and the region of the internal jugular vein are more
often involved and are usually indurated. He stated
that in 90 per cent. of the bodies examined the glands
showed streptococcus infection and 10 per cent. yielded
other bacteria. Kretz believes that many children suffer
from acute glandular fever, due to angina, and that the
infectious microörganisms pass rapidly through the
cervical lymph channels and glands with resulting severe
bacteriemia and fever. Hence a fatal result obtains in
virulent types of glandular fever in children. He states
that in older people the filtration through the deeper

cervical glands is slower. Consequently the virulence of the bacteria and the degree of bacteriemia may be less. The lymph node infection may disappear with the removal of the primary focus or may persist actively as new foci in the production of systemic disease or the infection of the nodes may become permanently latent.

Chronic Bronchitis and Bronchiectasis

Long standing bronchitis associated with emphysema, asthma, and bronchiectatic cavities presents a type of localized chronic infection which may be an etiologic factor in systemic infection and trophometabolic changes in bones and joints probably due to toxic products absorbed from the site of infection. The sputa in the conditions named yield cultures of many saprophytic bacteria as well as streptococci, staphylococci, pneumococci, influenza bacilli, micrococcus catarrhalis, fusiform anaerobes and other pathogenic bacteria.

Focal Infection of the Gastro-intestinal Canal, Vermiform Appendix, Gall-bladder and Pancreas

Auto-infection and auto-intoxication from the intestinal canal as a cause of disease is a popular idea with the medical profession. Stasis of the intestinal contents is alleged to be an important factor in the causation of auto-infection. Intestinal stasis may be due to habitual constipation, to partial obstruction of the intestines due to congenital defects, or to acquired morbid anatomical conditions which favor the presence of pathogenic bacteria with putrefactive changes, resulting, it is believed by many, in toxemia and systemic disease. Anemia, chronic arthritis, Bright's disease, arteriosclerosis, and even local diseases like appendicitis, cholecystitis calculosa and peptic ulcer, are believed to be caused by stasis and putrefactive changes in the intestinal contents. This large focus of infection has been attacked in the attempt to remove the offending bacteria by intestinal antiseptics, colonic flushing, buttermilk and other lactic acid bacilli containing fluids and tablets and cathartic waters, and the surgeon has invaded the abdomen to correct the intestinal stasis by removing kinks, veils and other alleged deformities, and even by resecting the entire colon.

There is doubtless some truth in the theory of intestinal infection, but the pathogenic microörganisms in the intestinal canal, which remain there as infectious organisms, gain entrance chiefly by swallowing infectious material from the mouth, throat and nose and also through infected food and drink, especially milk, for milk is very apt to contain streptococci which are virulent or may become so. Streptococci and other pathogenic bacteria probably infect the lymph tissue of the intestine or may pass into the lymph nodes of the mesentery and set up active or passive infection. As we shall see later, streptococcal infection from a focus in the head may hematogenously cause appendicitis, cholecystitis, peptic ulcer and pancreatitis. In addition to the immediate local damage, the bacteria in these tissues may form new foci from which proximal lymph nodes may become infected. From these new foci further extension of the infection may take place through the lymph channels or the blood stream or through both.

Appendicitis is usually caused by a strain of the streptococcus group from a mouth or throat focus. The colon bacilli and other members of the intestinal bacterial flora in the appendix may take on pathogenic qualities and cause a mixed infection. Often this mixed infection is fulminating and severe. Chronic types of appendicitis not only cause local distress and digestive disturbances, but may become a cause of infection of the mesenteric glands and through the lymph vessels and blood stream may infect the liver, bile tracts, and subdiaphragmatic tissues. Cholecystitis may also be caused by a streptococcus infection from a focus of the head. The infectious microörganism carried in the blood stream from the focus may lodge in the terminal blood vessels of the fundus of the gall-bladder. The inoculated blood vessel becomes wholly or partly occluded by endothelial proliferation and leukocytic infiltration, and blood containing the bacteria escapes into the wall of the bladder. Necrosis of the local tissues and rupture of the infected material into the gall-bladder may occur. Acute severe cholecystitis may result. Less severe infection may result in a chronic cholecystitis and subsequent gall-stone formation. Typhoid and colon bacilli may cause cholecystitis or may be associated in a mixed infection of the organ. Cholecystitis may be a focus of systemic infection.

The rectum, with its rich supply of hemorrhoidal veins, becomes a focus of infection, through ulcers, infected thrombi in veins and local abscesses. Infected thrombi from these points may produce acute circumscribed hepatitis (abscess), and bacteriemia.

Foci of Infection of the Genito-urinary Tract

Immediately after childbirth, miscarriage or abortion, the endometrium is very susceptible to infection by any of the pyogenic microörganisms. The resulting focus is usually serious because of the tendency to the formation of infected thrombi in the uterine sinuses. The bacteriemia which results is severe. At other times the endometrium is not a frequent site of focal infection.

The fallopian tubes are very susceptible to infection with pyogenic bacteria, but most frequently the cause is the gonococcus with resulting obliterating salpingitis or abscess which may infect the peritoneum. Tuberculous salpingitis may cause tuberculous peritonitis. Focal infection in the form of gonorrheal vaginitis is a common disease of defective girls and of girls in hospitals and public institutions. The condition is important because of the readiness with which it is conveyed from individual to individual by contact or through fomites. The condition usually remains a local one with consequent discomfort confined to the parts involved. Occasionally the peritoneum, joints and other tissues may become infected from the vaginal, uterine and tubal focus.

The seminal vesicles and testes are sites of focal infection with the gonococcus, tubercle bacillus and pyogenic bacteria.

Probably tuberculous infection of the genital apparatus is secondary to a focus elsewhere. Tuberculous infection of testes usually involves the seminal ducts and vesicles by extension through the lymph channels, blood stream or vas deferens. This focus may result in general tuberculosis or involve the urinary bladder and kidney by the blood stream or lymph canals.

Gonorrheal vesiculitis may be acute or chronic and lead to gonorrheal arthritis, acute or chronic, or to gonorrheal bacteriemia, and ulcerative endocarditis. Infection of the seminal vesicles may be due to streptococci and staphylococci and cause systemic disease. The prostate gland may be infected with gonococci, streptococci, staphylococci, tubercle bacilli, colon bacilli and other less important bacteria. When infected and enlarged it is an important factor in infection of the bladder, ureters and kidneys, by causing urinary obstruction and cystitis. Cystitis may be due to pyogenic bacteria, tubercle bacilli, bacillus pyocyaneus, typhoid bacilli and other bacteria. The colon bacillus is a very common inhabitant of the urinary tract and usually is apparently not harmful. In the presence of bladder stasis and in other types of cystitis (tuberculous, streptococcus, staphylococcus cystitis), the colon bacteria may take on pathogenic qualities as a mixed infection. Acute and chronic cystitis may be the source of infection of contiguous tissues and through the lymphatic vessels and lymph nodes of the base of the bladder and in the walls of the ureters, infection of the pelvis and parenchyma of the kidneys and perirenal tissues may occur as shown by S. Sugimura (4) and Carl Franke (5). The kidney and its pelvis, however, is usually infected hematogenously with pyogenic bacteria, typhoid, colon and tubercle bacilli and other microörganisms. Indeed cultures of the urine, with a proper technic, will yield characteristic bacteria, during the incidence of many infectious general and local diseases, as shown by George F. Dick and Gladys R. Dick (6). The kidney and renal pelvis may be the site of focal infection which may cause infection of the ureters and bladder through the urine contaminated with tubercle, colon, typhoid and pyocyaneus bacilli, pyogenic cocci, bacillus proteus and with other bacteria.

Subcutaneous abscesses and abscesses about the nails are occasionally the source of systemic infection. Furuncles and carbuncles are well known sources of acute bacteriemia, especially in patients debilitated by exhausting diseases of which diabetes mellitus is an example.

SUSCEPTIBILITY TO SYSTEMIC AND LOCAL DISEASES FROM THE FOCUS OF INFECTION

The high percentage of incidence of localized infection, especially about the head, has already been stated. The greater number of these individuals affected, both young and old, do not develop acute systemic disease therefrom. A majority of children suffer from chronic infection of the tonsils and nasopharyngeal lymphoid tissue with occasional acute exacerbations, while the incidence of acute rheumatic fever and endocarditis is relatively small in youth. Nevertheless, rheumatic fever and endocarditis are unquestionably the result of focal infection of the mouth and throat.

A majority of civilized mankind, who are city dwellers, carry a latent tuberculous focus, usually infected lymph nodes of the mediastinum, mesentery or elsewhere in the body. A comparatively small number develop clinically recognizable tuberculosis.

The marked prevalence of alveolar abscess is not associated with the frequent incidence of acute systemic infection. Probably the frequent relation of pyorrhea to rheumatic fever, heart disease, nephritis and other acute local and general infections has not been given the etiologic importance it deserves. Granting this fact one must still recognize the comparatively small incidence of acute systemic disease arising from alveolar abscess.

The incidence of chronic gonorrheal infection of the prostate gland, seminal vesicles, vagina and fallopian tubes is very large as compared with the occurrence of gonorrheal arthritis, tenovaginitis, gonococcemia, and ulcerative endocarditis.

The escape of a great majority of persons who harbor foci of infection from manifest clinical systemic disease, is the reason given by many thoughtful physicians for disbelief in the etiologic relation of foci of infection to systemic and local infection, especially of the chronic types.

Based upon the present knowledge obtained by clinical and laboratory research and experiments upon the lower animals, there can be no doubt now of the etiologic relation of localized infection to both acute and chronic systemic diseases. Many of the systemic chronic processes are sequential to primary acute diseases, etiologically related to focal infection. Other chronic systemic diseases are primarily due to infection derived from focal infection.

The relatively rare incidence of systemic disease as compared with the marked prevalence of focal infection may be answered, partially, at any rate, by well known facts concerning immunity both natural and acquired.

The natural defenses of the body, due to the bactericidal and antitoxic powers of the tissues, blood plasma and cells, especially the phagocytes, protect the majority of us from the acute infectious diseases. All individuals do not possess an equal degree of natural immunity; some more readily succumb to the invading infectious agents. When the animal body is invaded with pathogenic bacteria the natural defenses are increased by their presence in the tissues and blood. The processes are: first, the phenomenon of positive chemotaxis with resulting leukocytosis and the accumulation of leukocytes in the areas of infection of the tissues by the formation of local exudates, liquid (purulent) and fibrinoplastic, which may serve as walls of protection against further direct invasion; second, leukocytic phagocytosis with destruction of the invading bacteria; and third, the formation of protective antibodies in the blood and tissues.

Similar protective processes may be induced in the body by the injection of non-lethal amounts of living or of dead pathogenic bacteria into a healthy man or animal.

It is not improbable that the bacteria of a focal infection may excite the development of additional defenses in the host and prevent the evolution of a sequential systemic disease.

Bacteria may diminish in virulency and pathogenicity

and exist as harmless parasites of the skin, mucous membranes and probably also as foci in the tissues (Kolle and Wassermann (7)), for it is known that the reaction of the tissues is influenced by the virulence of the bacteria. A non-virulent streptococcus would be disposed of by the tissues with but little local or general reaction.

GREATER SUSCEPTIBILITY TO SYSTEMIC DISEASE FROM A FOCAL INFECTION UNDOUBTEDLY OCCURS

Immunity both natural and acquired as described is not absolute. Pasteur found that the marked immunity of the chicken to anthrax could be overcome by lowering the body temperature by immersion of the fowl in cold water. It is known that physical and mental exhaustion, starvation, exposure to cold, debility from alcoholic dissipation, the misuse of narcotic drugs and exhausting general disease may reduce the natural resistance.

Innumerable instances of the incidence of the sudden onset of pneumonia, rheumatic fever, tonsillitis, sinusitis, nephritis, septicemia and other infectious processes have been recorded after exposure to extreme cold. Undoubtedly the latent pathogenic bacteria usually present in the nose and throat may acquire coincidently with the exposure specific pathogenicity, and are able to invade the host because of the lowered resistance and because of added virulency. The acquisition of specific pathogenicity and tissue affinity by the members of the streptococcus-pneumococcus group will be fully considered.

Exhaustion and debility from physical and mental overwork, starvation, chronic disease and other conditions are important etiologic factors in the occurrence of acute and chronic systemic disease from focal infection. This is notably true of the chronic infectious arthritis and myositis.

Many of the lesser ills of the body in the form of subjective soreness of the tissues, joints, muscles and nerves are possibly the result of slight infection from a focus in the mouth or throat or some other region of the body, especially in individuals with a lessened resistance. This is perhaps a vague hypothesis, but instances of the disappearance of these clinical phenomena with the institution of individual hygiene and removal of an existing focus of infection is suggestive of the truth of the statement.

THE DIAGNOSIS OF THE FOCUS OF INFECTION

Usually a focus of infection is disregarded by the patient and physician unless it cause local discomfort. When a systemic disease occurs which present-day knowledge associates with a primary infectious focus, the site of the focus must be located. The character of the systemic disease may point to the most likely location of the primary portal of infection. The primary focus of acute rheumatic fever, endocarditis, chorea, myositis, glomerulonephritis, peptic ulcer, appendicitis and chronic deforming arthritis, as examples, is usually located in the head and usually in the form of alveolar abscesses, acute or chronic tonsillitis and sinusitis. One would look for the focus of gonorrheal arthritis in the genito-urinary tract. The failure to find a focus in the expected situation should indicate an extension of the field of examination until the primary infection shall have been found. In a superficial and hasty examination the site of the focus of infection may escape detection or the focus may be assumed to be in uninfected tissues and organs. Every patient should be carefully interrogated as to the past and present condition; a general examination should be made, including, if necessary, the services of specialists in diseases of the ear, nose and throat, the pelvic organs and the gastro-intestinal tract, and in all patients with evidence of pyorrhea and sinusitis the service of the röntgenologist is demanded. Bacterial cultures made from the surface of the gums and tonsils, which will usually yield pathologic types of bacteria, are not an index of focal infection located in the dental alveoli or tonsils. In alveolar abscess, by scraping the accumulated "tartar" and exudate from the exposed neck of the tooth and by penetrating as deeply as possible into the infected alveolus, one may readily obtain material for microscopic examination which usually yields endameba buccalis and bacteria. Cultures of the feces may yield strains of streptococci and other bacteria not usually found in the intestinal flora. These bacteria may not be specifically pathogenic in the intestinal habitat and if free in the intestinal contents and not infecting the intestinal structures are quite likely not to be harmful to the host. Bacteriological examination including cultures should always be made of the sputa, urine, uterine, vaginal and urethral discharges and exudates obtained by massage of the prostate gland and seminal vesicles, for they often yield results of diagnostic importance. The nature of the general disease and its relation to a supposed focus may be made more evident by the coincident histologic and bacteriologic studies, both miscroscopic and cultural, of exudates of synovial cavities, and of excised lymph nodes proximal to the infected regions; bits of infected muscles; fibrous nodes on tendons and aponeuroses; the blood, and also of the exudate of the focus; and by the inoculation of animals with strains of the dominant pathogenic bacteria so obtained, while the cultures are young. The discovery of the similarity of the pathogenic organisms in cultural characteristics, in the focus of infection and in the infected tissues, and the production of a similar infectious process in the inoculated animal from the tissues of which the infectious bacteria are afterwards recovered, constitute reasonable proof of the etiologic relation of the focus of infection to the existing systemic infection. Many successful clinical and laboratory studies of this kind have been made with patients suffering with rheumatic fever, subacute or chronic infectious endocarditis, chronic infectious arthritis, appendicitis, peptic ulcer, cholecystitis, glomerulonephritis and other diseases.

MODE OF DISSEMINATION OF BACTERIA AND TOXIC PRODUCTS FROM THE FOCUS OF INFECTION

Hematogenous

Systemic infection and intoxication from a primary focus is usually hematogenous. The bacteria may be compared with emboli loosened from the place of origin and carried in the blood stream to the smallest and often terminal blood vessels. If virulent and endowed with specific elective pathogenic affinity for the tissues in which they will lodge, and if *in sufficient number*, the invading bacteria will excite characteristic reactions in the infected tissues and a sequential train of morbid anatomical lesions. The evolution of the anatomical lesions and the clinical phenomena aroused thereby are dependent on the type and virulence of the bacteria, the character of the tissue and the function of the organ involved. The specific tissue reaction consists of a local inflammation with endothelial proliferation of the lining of the blood vessel with or without thrombosis; blocking of the blood vessels; hemorrhage into the immediate tissue; positive chemotaxis with resulting multiplication of the leukocytes and plasma cells in the infected area, or fibrinoplastic exudate with local connective tissue overgrowth.

Lymphogenous

The infectious microörganisms may also pass from the focus to other tissues through the lymph channels and lymph nodes. This may occur from the primary focus coincidentally with hematogenous systemic infection. Primary focal infection of the tonsils, nasopharyngeal tissue, the accessory sinuses and the mastoid cells is not infrequently associated with secondary infection of the lymphatic vessels and lymph nodes of the neck, sometimes extending to the mediastinal lymph nodes. The lymph nodes which drain areas of tissues which have been infected hematogenously from a primary focus may become infected and enlarged from the systemically infected areas as in infected joints, cholecystitis, appendicitis and infection about the pelvic organs.

The tissue reaction which occurs in infected lymph nodes varies in intensity with the virulency and character of the invading bacteria. Thus a varying degree of inflammation results in proliferation of the lymphoid cells with swelling and tenderness of the nodes. These secondary foci may continue as active depots of supply of bacterial infection to other tissues. If the invading bacteria of the lymph node are pyogenic and virulent, positive chemotaxis will result in the invasion of the infected gland with leukocytes and a circumscribed abscess may result. Lymph node infection with necrotic changes may rupture into or may cause infectious thrombophlebitis in a contiguous vessel and bacteriemia may result. In other instances the infection in the lymph node may be a protection by holding the invading organisms in a tissue environment which renders them latent and for the time harmless to the patient.

SYSTEMIC INTOXICATION

Systematic intoxication from a focus of infection is characteristic of the exotoxic bacteria. Diphtheria and tetanus are two examples of infectious disease in which the morbid tissue reactions are caused by soluble toxins excreted by the specific microörganisms in a focal area.

It has been assumed that focal infection due to microorganisms which produce endotoxins may cause systemic disturbances by dissemination of toxic substances from the focus. It is suggested that the toxic material may be formed by biochemical reactions excited by the microörganisms and the tissues and cellular exudate of the focus; also that autolysis of the dead microörganisms of the focus sets free the endotoxin. Hence it is said that morbid processes of a degenerative and metabolic character which may occur in many organs and in varying degrees of severity, are caused by toxins and toxic substances elaborated in a focus of infection.

Semmelweis, Klebs, Virchow, Pasteur, Lister and others proved long ago that virulent microörganisms are the cause of infectious disease. Modern bacteriology and clinical research are adding day by day incontestable proof that bacterial invasion and infection of tissue is the fundamental cause of many of the systemic diseases, which have been classed as toxic, metabolic or nutritional. A sequence of the fundamental and primary infection of tissue may create a morbid anatomy, disturbed function, malnutrition and in consequence secondary metabolic and degenerative changes. The endotoxin of the invading bacteria is set free in the blood and tissues and is a factor in the cellular reaction expressed in general infection by chill, fever, disturbed functions and altered metabolism and in local infection by cellular reaction and symptoms varying with the character of the invading bacteria, the anatomical lesions and disturbance of function of the tissue and organ involved.

FOCAL INFECTION AND ANAPHYLAXIS

Focal infection may be the cause of the condition known as anaphylaxis. The bacterial protein of the pathogenic microörganism of the focus may sensitize the body cells.

If a foreign protein gains entrance to the body parenterally, via the blood stream or the lymphatics, the animal body always responds to the parenteral introduction of the foreign protein by the production of specific antibodies to that foreign albumen. The formation of the specific antibodies requires a certain period of time. After this interval a second introduction of the same protein, again by a parenteral route, results in a union of the newly formed antibody with the antigen (foreign protein), which may excite' physical phenomena of an explosive character. These phenomena, the so-called anaphylactic shock, differ materially with various species of animals and with man. In man the typical phenomena may consist of bronchial spasm, urticaria, vasodilatation and fall of blood pressure, eosinophilia, physical weakness and arthropathy. In some individuals, urticaria or bronchial asthma may be the only expression of anaphylaxis.

Anaphylaxis has been studied as serum disease by Rosenau and Anderson (44), Park (47) and others. Von Pirquet (43), Weil (42), Meltzer (52) and Vaughan (45) have shown the relation of anaphylaxis to the symptom expression of infectious disease and to bronchial asthma. Theobald Smith (39), Auer and Lewis (46), Jobling, Petersen and Eggstein (53) and many others have reported the result of extensive research upon laboratory animals in the production of immunity and of anaphylaxis.

The relation of anaphylaxis to bronchial asthma, many dermatological lesions, gastro-intestinal symptoms, cardiovascular disturbance, especially arterial hypotension and other morbid conditions, of man, has not received the attention which its importance demands. Definite clinical evidence has been established of the etiologic relation of confined focal infection to anaphylaxis, in the form of bronchial asthma and other morbid conditions. The subject is not well understood, but is so important that it demands the cooperative research of the immunologist and clinician.

FOCAL INFECTION

LECTURE II

THE STREPTOCOCCUS-PNEUMOCOCCUS GROUP. TRANSMUTABILITY OF THE MEMBERS THEREOF. PATHOGENICITY AND SPECIFIC TISSUE AFFINITY OF TRANSMUTATION FORMS

TRANSMUTATION WITHIN THE MEMBERS OF THE STREPTO-COCCUS-PNEUMOCOCCUS GROUP

Recent coordinate research in clinical medicine and bacteriology, fortified by animal experimentation, has made more evident the etiologic relation of focal infection to systemic disease.

The main and fundamental principles which have been proved are:

· 1. The apparent confirmation of the transmutability of the members of the streptococcus-pneumococcus group in variations of morphology, cultural characteristics, biological reactions and also of general and special pathogenicity.

2. The acquisition of pathogenic elective tissue affinity by bacteria in foci of infection in culture media and serial animal passage.

In a clinical and bacteriological study of chronic infectious endocarditis Rosenow (8) and Billings (9) confirmed the report of Schottmüller (10) in the isolation from the blood during life of the patient of a pure culture of streptococcus viridans. Schottmüller (10) isolated a streptococcus from patients with chronic infectious endocarditis, which grew fine colonies on blood agar plates, was non-hemolyzing, but produced a greenish halo around the colonies. In consequence it was named streptococcus viridans and because of its low pathogenicity for animals it was also called streptococcus mitior. The streptococcus viridans, isolated from the blood of our eleven patients, was cultivated in various media and animals were inoculated with successive strains. The behavior of the strains obtained from all patients was the same. The end result was a pneumococcus of specific pathogenicity for animals in the production of pneumococcemia and pneumonia.

In consequence of these results the bacteriological diagnosis of our series of observed patients was chronic pneumococcus endocarditis. Rosenow soon recognized the fact that the bacteria studied were typical pneumococci and that transmutation of the original pure culture of streptococcus viridans had occurred in form, culture characteristics and in general and special pathogenic virulence for animals.

Since that time Rosenow (8) has apparently confirmed the transmutability of the members of the streptococcus group and that the property of transmutation is reversible within the members of this family. He says: "From this study the apparent position of the various members of the streptococcus group may be illustrated by the position of the fingers in a partially flexed hand, in which the hemolytic streptococcus occupies the position of the little finger, the pneumococcus the place of the index finger (the opposite extreme), streptococcus viridans (representing the group of more or less saprophytic, non-hemolyzing streptococci) the middle finger, the streptococci from rheumatism the ring finger, and streptococcus mucosus, having some of the properties of both pneumococci and streptococci, the thumb. In this grouping there is in general an increase in parasitism and virulence as we

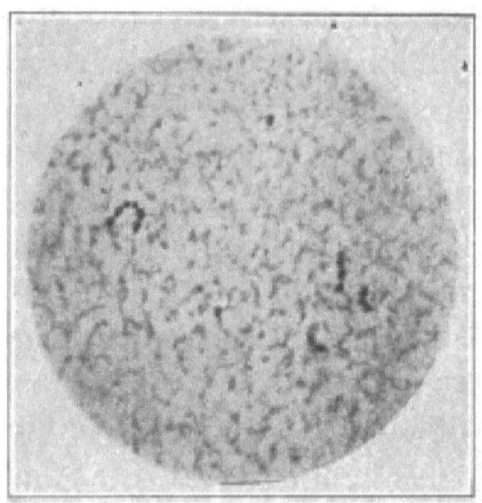

Fig. 1.—Strain 595 as a Hemolytic Streptococcus Isolated from a Case of Scarlet Fever. Smear from 24 hour culture in ascites-dextrose-broth. Gram stain.

approach the thumb (streptococcus mucosus)." Rosenow has arrived at this conclusion by working with strains of streptococci and pneumococci obtained from various sources: Strains of hemolytic streptococci isolated from patients suffering from erysipelas, puerperal sepsis, scarlatina, acute tonsillitis and acute polyarthritis; from cow's milk and other sources; strains of streptococcus viridans isolated from tonsils, alveolar abscesses, the blood, from other tissues and cow's milk; streptococcus mucosus from sputa, tonsils and else-

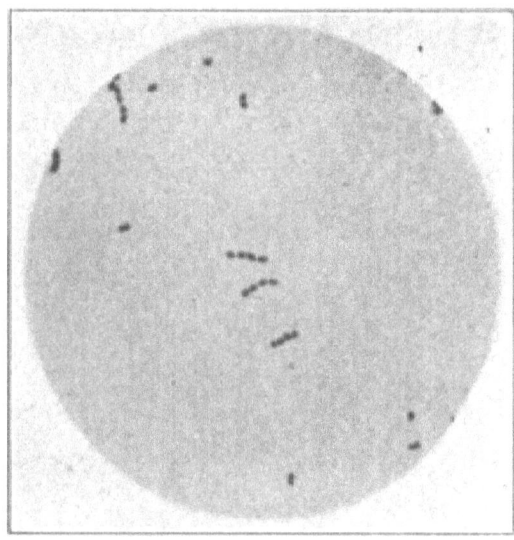

Fig. 2.—Strain 595 as Streptococcus Viridans. Smear from 24 hour culture in ascites-dextrose-broth. Gram stain.

where and pneumococci isolated from sputa, the blood during life and post mortem, the exudate of empyema, from hepatized lung and also Cole's (11) strains I and

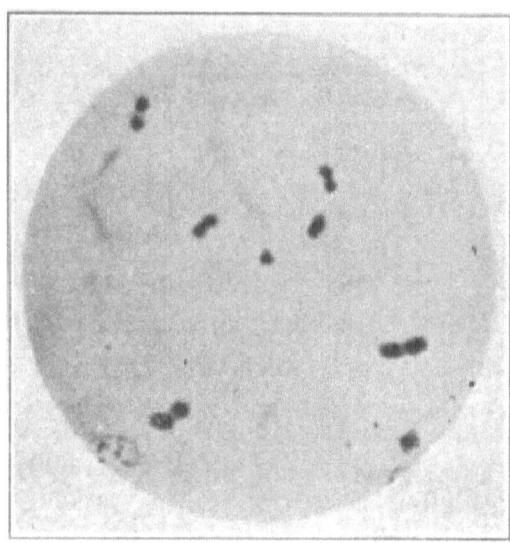

Fig. 3.—Strain 595 as a Pneumococcus. Smear from 24 hour culture in ascites-dextrose-broth. Capsule stain.

II. These have been successfully made to assume the varying types as to form, cultural characteristics, biologic reactions and special and general pathogenic virulence of the group.

The technic which Rosenow pursues consists of the use of the ordinary solid and liquid culture media in which the oxygen content is increased and decreased,

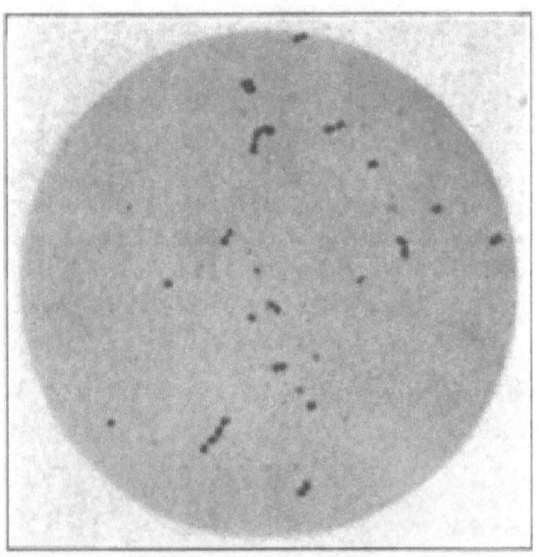

Fig. 4.—Strain of Streptococcus from Rheumatism Which Produced Slight Hemolysis on Blood Agar and Myositis in Animals. Smear from blood agar slant. Capsule stain.

the use of hypotonic and hypertonic media, cultures made in symbiosis with bacillus subtilis as the occasion may indicate and of serial animal inoculation. Haessli (12) produced transmutation of a non-color-forming strain of streptococcus fecalis, by passing it several times through horse serum, when it finally became strongly hemolytic and had acquired all the pathogenic characteristics of streptococcus erysipelas. By the same method streptococcus viridans first lost its greenish

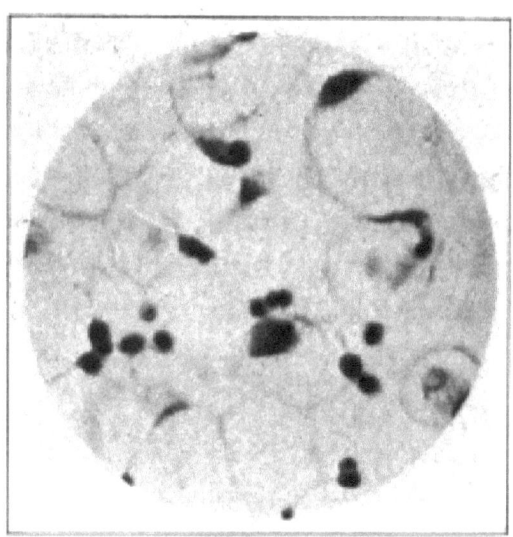

Fig. 5.—The Same Strain as in Fig. 4 After It Was Transformed Into a Pneumococcus. Smear from blood agar slant. Capsule stain.

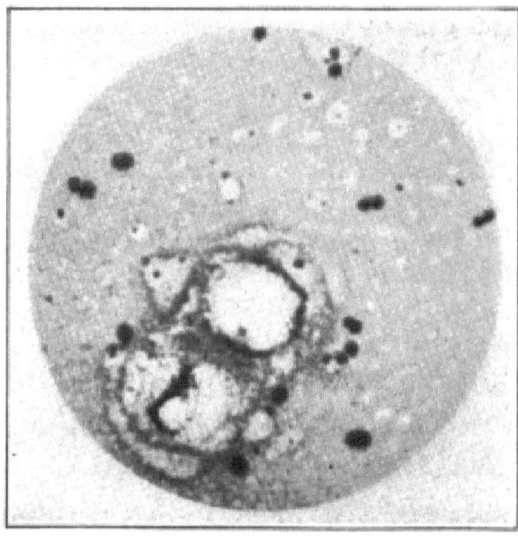

Fig. 6.—Highly Virulent Pneumococcus. Type 1. Originally Isolated by Neufeld. Smear from surface and water of condensation of blood agar slant. Capsule stain.

color producing quality, finally became hemolytic and a strain of streptococcus mucosus became hemolytic. Haessli finally states that his experiments confirm the clinical differentiation of streptococci as demonstrated by Schottmüller. Schottmüller (10) probably recognized the transmutability of members of the streptococcus group pathogenic for man which he classified as

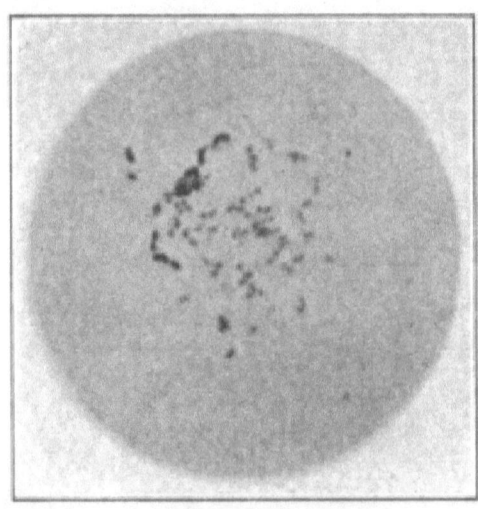

Fig. 7.—The Same Strain as in Fig. 6 After Transformation Into Hemolytic Streptococcus. Smear from surface and water of condensation of blood agar slant. Capsule stain.

streptococcus longus (hemolysans), streptococcus mitior (viridans) and streptococcus mucosus. Schottmüller (10) also described strains of streptococcus mucosus, which possessed all the characteristics of strains first isolated from patients with parametritis in 1896, obtained in pure culture from the blood and hepatized lung of five patients with clinical lobar pneumonia. The strains described occurred as diplococci with capsule in chains of ten to fourteen pairs. Evidently he did not recognize the pneumococcus as a member of the group and especially its close relation to the streptococcus mucosus. Transmutation within the members of other groups of pathogenic bacteria probably occurs. The members of the colon-typhoid group shade into one another in form, motility, cultural characteristics and in degrees of pathogenicity from nil to exalted virulence.

Virulence and Elective Pathogenic Tissue Affinity

The varying virulence of facultative pathogenic bacteria has been long recognized. Environment seems to play an important rôle. This seems especially true of living tissue environment. Not only may there be a variation in general virulence, but apparently a special pathogenic virulence for certain tissues may be acquired. In this connection we may note the recent epidemics of septic tonsillitis, frequently associated with fatal bacteriemia, due to milk infected with streptococci from human carriers. The acquirement of a selective specific tissue affinity by a strain of streptococci has been noted by Forssner (13). By culture in kidney and kidney extract the ordinary streptococcus pyogenes (hemolysans), which had no pathogenic elective affinity for the kidney, was converted into a strain, which injected intravenously into animals constantly produced outspoken anatomical lesions of the kidney. This Forssner believes is positive proof that the bacteria of a local infection may attain a specific pathogenic and elective tissue affinity.

By making continued cultures in bouillon, for a long time these specific kidney strains assumed a general virulence. Again grown on kidney and kidney extract, the specific kidney pathogenicity was regained and maintained through numberless generations. This specific kidney pathogenicity was lost after a few generations in continued bouillon cultures. The general virulence was also finally lost.

Poynton and Paine (14) in a discussion of the relation of malignant to rheumatic endocarditis state that the diplococcus isolated from patients with acute rheumatism caused acute non-suppurative arthritis and simple rheumatic endocarditis in rabbits. In culture after a few months the same strain of diplococci caused malignant endocarditis in the inoculated animal. They could not recover the diplococcus from the nodular vegetations in rheumatic endocarditis, but succeeded in obtaining pure cultures of a smaller diplococcus from the large vegetations and contained thrombi of malignant endocarditis. They concluded that the diplococcus rheumaticus was capable of producing not only arthritis and rheumatic endocarditis but also malignant endocarditis. Rationally we may interpret their observations and results as a transmutation of the diplococcus rheumaticus in virulency and in specific pathogenicity. Our clinical observations and Rosenow's experiments seem to show that the members of the streptococcus-pneumococcus group may acquire specific pathogenic elective affinity for certain tissues in the primary focus and also in the tissues.

Clinical examples have been observed of acute appendicitis; cholecystitis; acute gastric and duodenal ulcer; acute and subacute glomerulonephritis; rheumatic fever; erythema nodosum; herpes zoster; malignant endocarditis; simple endocarditis; myocarditis and other acute and chronic systemic diseases, associated with coincident focal infection of the tonsils, accessory sinuses, dental alveoli, the skin and its appendages, the fallopian tubes, the prostate and seminal vesicles and other foci. Dominant pathogenic bacteria have been isolated from tissues and exudates of patients at surgical operation; by blood culture; from the urine; from joint exudates and pieces of tissue (muscular, lymphoid, joint capsules and fibrous nodes), removed with the consent and often at the request of patients. These cultures have been intravenously injected into laboratory animals and at the same time cultures of bacteria isolated from the primary foci of the patients have been likewise used to inoculate other animals.

The evidences of the specific elective tissue affinity of the pathogenic streptococci from the various tissues and likewise of the primary foci is very marked. This is significantly expressed in the following table prepared by Rosenow (8) from an enormous number of animal experiments.

The principles of localized infection in man and animals are so important that the technic of the experiments and the interpretation of the table by Rosenow are quoted very fully here.

Technic

The streptococci were usually grown from sixteen to twenty-four hours at 37° C. in tall columns of ascites (10 per cent.) dextrose (0.2 per cent.) broth (0.6 + to 0.8 +) to which sterile tissue (guinea-pig kidney or heart muscle) was often added; the sterility of the ascites fluid and broth containing

ELECTIVE LOCALIZATION OF STREPTOCOCCI

Source of Streptococci		Strains (230)	Animals Injected (833)	Percentage of Animals Showing Lesions in																	
				Appendix	Stomach Hemor.	Duodenum Ulcer	Gall-bladder	Pancreas	Intestines	Joints	Endocardium	Pericardium	Myocardium	Muscles	Kidney	Lung	Skin	Tongue	Eye	Parotid
Appendicitis	When isolated	14	68	68	6	1	1	0	9	29	21	0	9	12	0	0	0	0	3	0
	Later	8	26	15	19	15	4	0	0	22	19	0	12	23	0	0	0	0	0	0
	After animal passage	7	22	45	45	30	40	0	20	36	20	4	20	25	10	0	0	0	0	0
Ulcer of stomach in man	When isolated	18	103	2	60	60	20	3	7	16	12	0	5	0	5	5	0	0	0	0
	Later	8	22	0	5	0	5	0	0	18	14	0	0	0	0	15	2	0	0	0
	After animal passage	7	39	0	23	33	30	15	15	21	5	0	3	3	8	5	0	0	0	0
Cholecystitis	When isolated	12	41	14	29	15	60	5	17	17	10	0	2	7	5	6	2	0	0	0
	Later	5	14	0	28	14	7	0	0	21	14	0	0	0	7	4	0	0	0	0
	After animal passage	5	16	8	31	13	56	19	13	25	19	0	13	0	13	0	0	0	0	0
Rheumatic fever	When isolated	24	71	0	23	18	3	3	3	66	45	27	44	27	39	21	6	0	0	0
	Later	8	14	21	14	21	0	0	0	21	21	32	28	16	21	5	0	0	10	0
	After animal passage	5	14	0	37	21	5	21	5	37	53	10	37	35	42	0	0	0	11	0
Erythema nodosum	When isolated	4	20	0	10	0	0	0	0	20	20	7	0	0	10	43	90	15	5	0
	Later	3	9	0	22	0	11	0	5	11	11	11	14	50	0	21	22	0	0	0
	After animal passage	6	14	10	21	8	50	13	7	50	14	7	5	11	7	20	43	15	15	0
Herpes zoster	When isolated	11	61	0	29	7	16	42	8	11	5	11	20	40	5	43	70	14	13	0
	Later	6	15	0	13	10	7	12	1	60	7	0	0	28	7	21	7	0	0	0
	After animal passage	4	7	15	28	5	0	7	0	43	0	14	37	3	0	20	28	0	0	0
Mumps	When isolated	9	19	12	21	10	21	42	10	42	15	0	12	12	5	43	15	15	8	73
	Later	5	8	0	4	5	0	12	12	24	24	0	35	75	2	15	12	14	0	24
Myositis	When isolated	8	40	2	7	10	2	7	7	20	10	4	20	0	20	20	7	0	8	0
Endocarditis	When isolated	5	44	0	17	0	5	0	15	15	64	0	15	7	7	7	2	0	0	0
Miscellaneous	When isolated	34	41	3	17	0	4	0	4	17	20	0	15	7	7	0	0	0	0	0
"Lab." strains	Before and after animal passage	5	100	2	18	5	2	2	2	45	49	0	15	12	10	17	2	0	6	0
Average percentage of animals injected with non-specific strains showing lesions in individual organs				5	20	9	11	6	8	27	14	2	10	12	9	11	2	1	3	0

NOTE. This table was used in a lantern slide to illustrate Lecture II. Since the lectures were delivered Rosenow has used the table in an article on Elective Localization of Streptococci, *Jour. A.M.A. LXVI, 1916, 1687.*

the tissue was always proved beforehand. After incubation smears were made, the cultures were centrifuged in the containers in which they were cultivated,[1] the supernatant fluid was decanted and the sediment suspended in sodium chlorid solution so that 1 c.c. of the suspension contained the growth from 15 c.c. of broth. The doses for rabbits (ear vein) were usually from 0.5 to 3 c.c., and for dogs (leg vein) from 1 to 5 c.c. of this suspension. The injections were made quite rapidly through a rather fine needle (22 gauge), usually within an hour after the suspension was made. Blood agar plate cultures were made at the time the suspensions were injected to study the character of the organisms, to test their viability and to save them for further study. This is an important precaution because negative results have at times proved to be due to early death of the recently isolated organisms in the broth cultures. In the accompanying table, "when isolated" indicates the first or second and, occasionally, the third or fourth cultures, or the first culture after one animal passage. "Later" indicates that the strains were cultivated for a week or longer. "After animal passage" indicates usually from the second to the sixth animal passage.

The strains tested from appendicitis, ulcer of the stomach, cholecystitis, rheumatic fever, erythema nodosum, myositis and endocarditis include strains isolated from the characteristic lesions as well as from the apparent atrium of infection. Those from herpes zoster were from the tonsils and spinal fluid, and those from epidemic parotitis were obtained by catheterizing Steno's duct and from the tonsils. The strains from miscellaneous sources were usually from tonsils approaching the normal condition; and the laboratory strains were streptococci or pneumococci cultivated on artificial mediums for a long time and had lost all apparent virulence. The figures in the lowest line of the table represent the average percentage incidence

[1] The common 8-ounce nursing bottle is used both as a culture flask and centrifugal tube, and serves the purpose admirably.

of lesions in individual organs following injection of various strains of streptococci except those from the specific disease. Thus the first figure indicates that 5 per cent. of the animals, injected with the various strains except those from appendicitis, showed lesions in the appendix.

Care was exercised to obtain growths from the depths of the supposed primary focus with as little contamination from the surface as possible, the cultures being made from the material expressed from the tonsils or from emulsion of extirpated tonsils after thorough washing in sodium chlorid solution. The material from the depths of pyorrheal pockets was obtained by means of a pipet.

For the study of pathogenicity of the cultures, dogs and rabbits were chiefly used, being killed with chloroform at the desired time, usually in from twenty-four to forty-eight hours. Post mortem examinations were always made as soon after death as possible. A thorough inspection in a bright light with the unaided eye or with the aid of a hand lens was made for focal lesions. The exact character of the lesions and the presence of the streptococci in each of the various diseases have been determined by microscopic study of sections. Cloudy swelling is not included in the results given in the table. Hemorrhage, localized necrosis, exudation and infiltration were the usual lesions. Thus, in case of the joints, hemorrhage about the joint or turbidity of fluid, as determined with a pipet, or both, were considered as evidence of arthritis. Hemorrhages in the pericardium and turbidity of pericardial fluid, due to leukocytes, were considered as evidence of pericarditis. The post mortem study of animals often symptomless is essential to obtain accurate knowledge of the pathogenicity of a culture, and must supplant the older method of merely finding out whether a culture produces death or not, a method still too much in vogue. The table includes data only from those animals in which the post mortem was comprehensive, and does not include some of the earlier experiments, especially on endocarditis. Increase in mortality rate, earlier death and greater degree and distribution of lesions following standard dosage were considered as proof of high virulence. Changes in the spleen and liver were so rare following injection of the strains as isolated, except those from cholecystitis, that they are not included in the table. Acute splenitis and such changes in the liver as focal necrosis, parenchymatous and bile duct hemorrhages and acute degeneration with marked acidity occurred, however, after the strains had acquired greater virulence from animal passage. In the earlier experiments not sufficient attention was paid to the occurrence of lesions in the thyroid, thymus, suprarenals and lymphatic glands. Later a closer search for lesions in these structures was made, especially after it was found that lesions in the thyroid followed intravenous injection of bacteria isolated from goiter. It must be said, too, that strains of streptococci from rheumatic fever, myositis and cholecystitis produce hemorrhages in the thyroid quite commonly, while those from other sources rarely produce them.

Results

A study of the table shows that streptococci from the various diseases often have a most striking affinity or tropism for the organs or tissues from which they are isolated. Thus, fourteen strains from appendicitis produced lesions in the appendix in 68 per cent. of the sixty-eight rabbits injected, which is in marked contrast to an average of only 5 per cent. (given in lowest line of table) of lesions in the appendix in the animals injected with the strains as isolated from sources other than appendicitis. Eighteen strains from ulcer of the stomach or duodenum produced hemorrhages in 60 per cent. and ulcer of the stomach or duodenum in 60 per cent., a combined total of 74 per cent. of the 103 animals injected, in contrast to an average of 20 per cent. hemorrhages and 9 per cent. ulcer following injection of other strains. Twelve strains from cholecystitis produced lesions in the gall-bladder in 80 per cent. of the forty-one animals injected, in contrast to an average incidence of lesions here of only 11 per cent. with the other strains. Twenty-four strains from rheumatic fever produced arthritis in 66 per cent., endocarditis in 46 per cent., pericarditis in 27 per cent., and myocarditis in 44 per cent. of the seventy-one animals injected, in contrast to an average of arthritis in 27 per cent., endocardial lesions in 14 per cent., pericarditis in 2 per cent. and myocarditis in 10 per cent. of the animals injected with strains from sources other than rheumatic fever. Six strains from erythema nodosum produced lesions of the skin in 90 per cent. of twenty animals injected, in contrast to an average of 2 per cent. in the animals injected with the strains from sources other than erythema nodosum and herpes zoster. Eleven strains from herpes zoster produced herpetiform lesions of the skin, lips, tongue or conjunctivae in 77 per cent. of the sixty-one animals injected, in contrast to the average of only 1 per cent. of what seemed to be herpes of the skin with the other strains. Nine strains of streptococcal organisms from epidemic parotitis produced lesions in one or both parotid glands in 73 per cent. of the nineteen animals injected intravenously, in contrast to no instance of lesions here with the other strains. Three strains from cases of true myositis produced myositis in 75 per cent. and myocarditis (chiefly of the right ventricle) in 35 per cent. of the forty animals injected, in contrast to an average of myositis of 12 per cent. and myocarditis of 10 per cent. following injection of strains from sources other than myositis or rheumatic fever and eight strains of streptococcus viridans from chronic septic endocarditis produced lesions in the endocardium in 84 per cent. of the forty-four animals injected, in contrast to an average of 15 per cent. with the strains other than those from endocarditis. The results following injection of the miscellaneous strains (usually the first culture from tonsils) and the laboratory strains serve as a basis of comparison with those following injection of the strains from the various diseases, and correspond roughly with the total average incidence of lesions in the various organs as given in the lowest line of the table.

While the incidence of lesions in the organs following injection of the strains isolated from such organs is high, as shown by these figures, the appearances at the necropsy are even more significant. In many instances in which the animals survive the injection for some time, no other focal lesions could be found except those in the organ in question; and when the animal died early, these lesions were the marked feature and the associated ones were relatively insignificant. Frequently the injection of a very small dose was sufficient to prove the elective localization. This elective property was shown not only by the cultures from tissues and foci but also by the bacteria contained in the foci, directly injected in other animals.

In many cases of both acute and chronic diseases the apparent atrium of infection was found to harbor streptococci having elective affinity; in the former usually only at the time of the attack, in the latter in some instances for months. The elective affinity, however, was less marked in the strains isolated from the supposed focus than in the strains isolated from the lesions in the various organs. The rather wide range of lesions, as indicated in the table, following the injection of the strains from herpes zoster and parotitis is due to the fact that often primary mixed cultures from tonsils and pyorrheal pockets were injected.

Attempts to find a method which would preserve the original tropic property, while only partially successful, have shown that it may be preserved for some weeks in the deeper colonies of the original shake cultures and for as long as seven months by keeping the suspensions containing sterile tissue in the ice chest, thus maintaining the bacteria in a condition of latent life.

The localization of the strains from appendicitis, ulcer of the stomach and cholecystitis as isolated, after cultivation and after animal passage, is of particular interest. It should be stated here, however, that these strains resemble one another very closely indeed in cultural and other respects. Those from appendicitis are the least virulent, those from ulcer occupy a middle position and those from cholecystitis are the most virulent. The virulence seems to be one of the factors that determine their place of survival after intravenous injection. Now if the localization is dependent to a certain extent on virulence, then the occurrence of ulcer and cholecystitis should become greater as the strains from the appendix are passed through animals, and appendicitis should occur oftener after the strains from ulcer and cholecystitis lose virulence from cultivation on artificial mediums. This is found actually to be the case (see figures in table). In this connection other facts should be mentioned. None of the strains from appendicitis produced pancreatitis. The strains from ulcer and cholecystitis as isolated (mostly those from acute cases) produced pancreatitis in 3 per cent. and 5 per cent., respectively, of the animals injected. After animal passage, pancreatitis occurred in 15 and 19 per cent. respectively, while after cultivation on artificial mediums pancreatitis in no case was obtained.

Lesions in the intestines, exclusive of the duodenum, were more common with the strains from cholecystitis and rheumatism than with those from appendicitis, and all the strains produced intestinal lesions (chiefly of the mucous membrane and lymphoid structures) quite commonly after they had been passed through animals, whereas, after cultivation for a time, no noteworthy lesions were found in the intestinal tract.

The streptococci studied from parotitis resemble the organism described by Herb[1] and, like hers, produced the characteristic picture of mumps in dogs when injected into Steno's duct. Intravenous injection of these organisms produced marked edema and hemorrhage in and surrounding the parotid. The affinity was so great that the streptococci were found in

[1] Herb, Isabella C.: Experimental Parotitis, Arch. Int. Med., September, 1909, p. 201.

pure culture in the enlarged parotid in three of five full-time puppies removed from the uterus of a dog which was chloroformed during a marked parotitis following injection into Steno's duct. Antigens prepared from a number of these strains were found to bind specifically complement in serum from parotitis (Howell).

Lesions in the skeletal muscles occurred in 75 per cent. of the animals injected. The number of lesions in the muscles and myocardium in the animals injected with strains from myositis was often in proportion to the quantity injected, and occurred mostly in the tendinous portion and in the right ventricle.

Lesions in the kidney were especially common after injections of streptococci from rheumatic fever (39 per cent.) and from endocarditis (20 per cent.). These occurred chiefly in the medullary portion in the former and in the glomeruli in the latter.

Lesions in the lung, consisting usually of hemorrhages and edema, were rare following injection of the strains when isolated and after they were cultivated on artificial mediums but, just as was found previously, they occurred oftener after the virulence was increased by animal passage.

That the streptococci are the underlying cause of the diseases from the lesions of which they were isolated is indicated further by the fact that they have elective affinity for the corresponding structures in animals. Moreover, the fact that the same streptococcus may be made to localize in different organs is in consonance with the knowledge that streptococci may cause diseases with different symptomatology. The possibility, however, that they are secondary invaders to some ultramicroscopic, filterable organism has to be considered. Filtrates of the streptococcal cultures from various diseases were injected in the organs from which the strains were isolated; the lesions, however, were not due to living organisms because the broth which was inoculated and incubated with the tissues failed to produce any lesions. The results, while inconclusive, may be said to indicate that streptococci produce substances which cause injury specifically in the tissues from which the strains are isolated.

*　　*　　*　　*　　*　　*　　*　　*　　*

Although the circulation is an important factor in determining localization, the tissues themselves play an even more important rôle. The question whether the lesions in the organ for which a particular strain appears to have elective affinity are due to the lodgment of a larger number of bacteria here than in the other organs, or whether the bacteria lodged in equal numbers in the various organs but survive only in the one showing lesions, is now under study. The evidence already obtained, however, points strongly to the former mechanism. It appears that the cells of the tissues for which a given strain shows elective affinity take the bacteria out of the circulation as if by a magnet—adsorption.

This remarkable tropic condition tends to disappear quite promptly both on cultivating the streptococci on artificial mediums and on passing them successively through animals, and this may occur without demonstrable changes in morphology, grouping or character of chain formation. I have previously shown that the ability of streptococcus viridans and staphylococci to produce lesions in the endocardium is due partly to physical clumping. A careful study of smears of the suspensions injected in these experiments revealed no constant relation between localization and clumping or size of the bacteria.

Individual variations in resistance to infection were found in the injected animals. The effects of these conditions in the host as determining factors in localization are important; they are probably expressions of differences in metabolism, oxidation rates, etc., which influence the soil for bacteria. The tendency of virulent bacteria, temporarily or permanently, to render this soil less favorable for their growth is well established. There is some evidence, on the other hand, which goes to show that certain bacteria of very low virulence (commonly found in chronic foci of infection) tend actually to make this soil more favorable. But it must be considered that differences in the host may afford the peculiar type of reaction, or that the individual harbors a particular form of focus of infection which is favorable for bacteria to acquire elective properties. The following facts support the latter view: (1) the common occurrence of certain non-contagious diseases, such as herpes zoster, ulcer of the stomach, etc., during definite age periods; (2) the fact that foci of infection afford opportunity for bacteria to grow under varying grades of oxygen pressure and in mixed culture, both of which have been shown to cause changes in virulence and other properties of bacteria, including the streptococcus group; (3) the occurrence of systemic infections such as rheumatic fever, appendicitis, ulcer of the stomach, etc., usually after the acute symptoms in follicular tonsillitis (hemolytic streptococci) have subsided, and (4) the finding in the focus and involved tissues at the time of the systemic infection, streptococci having elective affinity for these structures in animals.

Since different bacteria may acquire simultaneously affinity for the same tissue, diseases which resemble each other more or less closely, such as the different forms of arthritis, may be due to bacteria of different species each having elective affinity for the particular structures involved.

The figures in the lowest line of the table represent the results of numerous experiments (833) with streptococci (220) from a wide range of sources, and may therefore be regarded as an index of the liability of the various organs to infection. Thus, joint lesions occurred more often (27 per cent.) than lesions in other organs, corresponding to the frequent occurrence of spontaneous arthritis in man and animals. The occurrence of lesions in the stomach (20 per cent.), valves of the heart (14 per per cent.), myocardium (12 per cent.) and skeletal muscles (12 per cent.) correspond in a general way to the occurrence of infection in these organs in man. The very infrequent involvement of the skin, tongue and the parotid in the animals is in keeping with the rarity of embolic infections in these structures. The character of the lesions and their occurrence simultaneously in the joints, heart, muscles and kidneys, and the development of chorea (7 per cent. mostly in young rabbits) following injection of the streptococci from rheumatic fever, parallels quite closely the phenomena of rheumatic infection as observed in man. The strains from erythema nodosum resemble those from rheumatic fever, producing a relatively high incidence of arthritis, pericarditis and myositis, a fact which supports the view held by clinical observers, that the causative agents of rheumatic fever and erythema nodosum must be similar.

The tendency to localize electively within a limited range, "monotropism," is most highly developed in the relatively non-virulent strains isolated from chronic lesions. In the more virulent strains from acute lesions and after animal passage, this tendency is less highly developed, the lesions occurring over a wider range, "polytropism." Since the bacteria which have grown in a given tissue acquire greater affinity for this tissue, the likelihood of these bacteria to involve other structures is relatively slight; hence the secondary focus, a cholecystitis, for example, would appear to be less important as a distributer of bacteria than the primary focus; if, however, the secondary focus happens to be in a joint, of which there are many, it may play an important rôle in causing extension to uninvolved joints and in preventing recovery.

The great importance of the enormous and painstaking experiments and the rational deductions made by Rosenow must be apparent to clinicians, bacteriologists and pathologists.

The practical application of the principles involved may serve to lessen the incidence of and the recrudescence of many local inflammatory organic diseases, notably appendicitis, ulcer of the stomach and duodenum, cholecystitis, glomerulonephritis, acute and chronic arthritis and other abnormal conditions, by the removal of the primary focal cause.

LECTURE III

ACUTE DISEASES RELATED TO FOCAL INFECTION

We have considered the causes, character and diagnosis of focal infection; the mode of systemic infection from the focus; the important fact of transmutation within the members of the streptococcus-pneumococcus group, with coincident variations of specific pathogenicity and virulency and the acquirement of pathogenic elective tissue affinity by bacteria in culture media, in serial animal passage and in the foci of infection.

We may now understandingly consider some of the systemic infections which are etiologically related to focal infection.

ACUTE RHEUMATIC FEVER

It is not necessary to consider the controversies which have taken place concerning the bacterial cause of rheumatic fever. There is now no doubt that the diplococcus also called by other observers micrococcus rheumaticus and streptococcus rheumaticus, isolated from the blood and joint fluids, throat and endocardial nodes of patients suffering from rheumatic fever by Poynton and Paine (14) confirmed by Beattie (15), Walker and Ryffel (16) and finally and conclusively by Rosenow (8), is the true infectious cause of the disease.

With a knowledge of the possibility of transmutation in form, cultural characteristics and coincident variation in specific pathogenicity, virulency and tissue affinity, we may now understand the conflicting results of animal inoculation with undifferentiated strains of streptococci as reported by many workers. It is a well known fact that virulent strains of streptococci, when injected intravenously into animals, may produce acute arthritis, usually with such violent tissue reaction that suppuration occurs. But the streptococcus rheumaticus never produces suppuration. Doubt of its etiologic relation to acute rheumatism also arose from the fact that it was not usually found by cultural methods in the joint exudate and circulating blood of patients. But Rosenow (8) has found that with an improved technic it may be always found, at the proper stage of the disease, in the joint exudate, joint capsule, circulating blood, tonsil, alveolar abscess or other focus.

Rosenow's studies of cultures from the joint exudate of patients with acute rheumatism yielded three strains. From five patients without muscular involvement, on blood agar the colonies were green and grew in long chains, longer than streptococcus viridans. Injected intravenously into animals they developed acute non-destructive arthritis, myositis, marked myocarditis with endocarditis and occasionally pericarditis. From six patients with acute rheumatic fever involving the joints and muscles the isolated microörganisms produced slight hazy hemolysis on blood agar, and grew as diplococci in the short chains. Injected intravenously the inoculated animals developed non-destructive, acute arthritis, myositis, severe myocarditis, endocarditis and occasionally pericarditis. From three patients with acute rheumatism the joint exudate yielded small gray colonies on blood agar. They grew in clumps of small micrococci and diplococci and occasionally in short chains. Animals injected intravenously developed a characteristic arthritis with endocarditis and pericarditis, but no myositis or myocarditis.

The three types of cocci found by Rosenow explains the variations in name given by Poynton, Paine, Walker and Beattie, i. e.: diplococcus, streptococcus and micrococcus rheumaticus.

The virulence of all the strains is low. All are very sensitive to oxygen pressure in culture and all multiply at low temperature. The three strains are transmutable. All produce excessive acidity in dextrose broth. Walker and Ryffel (16) found formic acid in the cultures of the strains with which they worked.

Exposure of the inoculated animal to low temperature intensifies the disease, presumably by lowering phagocytosis and by vasocontraction. Rosenow also noted in some injected animals the development of iritis by hematogenous infection. Some inoculated animals also developed appendicitis, colitis, mesenteric lymphadenitis and diarrhea. Poynton and Paine (14) also have noted the occurrence of obscure infection of intestines and appendix of animals intravenously inoculated with the diplococcus rheumaticus. The intestinal lesions produced in animals and the fact that the stool of a patient with rheumatic fever may yield cultures of streptococcus rheumaticus indicate that the intestinal tract and mesenteric lymph nodes may be a secondary and possibly a primary focus of rheumatic fever.

Rosenow has shown that cultures kept for one to eight months lose the power to grow at a low temperature, the sensitiveness to oxygen tension, the production of excessive acid in dextrose broth and at the same time lose the specific pathogenic affinity for joint, muscle, myocardium, endocardium and pericardium. By serial animal passage the streptococcus rheumaticus and especially the diplococcus type, may assume an affinity for the appendix, stomach and gall-bladder.

The clinical and bacteriological research of Poynton and Paine, the use of blood agar media by Schottmüller to differentiate members of the streptococcus group which are pathogenic for man, and the confirmatory work of Rosenow have proven conclusively the character of the infectious microörganism which causes rheumatic fever with arthritis, myositis, endocarditis, myocarditis, pericarditis and pleuritis.

Rheumatic fever occurs most frequently in the temperate zone, among people who live under conditions which are unhealthful and which especially induce focal infection. It is most prevalent in the young and in the more exposed male of all ages. The excess of lymphoid tissue in the pharynx and nose of the young explains the frequency of the incidence of the focal infection and the subsequent rheumatism. The frequent association of the onset of rheumatic fever with lowering of the body temperature by exposure to cold and a wetting is explained by the increased specific virulency of the bacterial cause acquired by a low tem-

perature and the coincident lessened resistance of the
patient due to the exposure. The frequent absence of
evidence of acute focal infection at the onset of the
systemic disease is not an evidence that no focus exists.
The latent chronic streptococcus infection of tonsillitis,
pyorrhea alveolaris, sinusitis, etc., may suddenly acquire
increased virulence and specific pathogenic affinity with
varying degrees of focal tissue reaction. This transmutation of type and pathogenicity certainly occurs in the
focus of infection. The removal of the tonsils and other
sites of focal infection has been followed by complete
recovery of prolonged, subacute and chronic types
of arthritis and has unquestionably prevented recurrent
attacks of rheumatic fever to which the susceptibility
is increased by one or more attacks. The occurrence of
rheumatic fever after the removal of an apparent focus
may be due to secondary systemic latent foci in lymph
nodes proximal to joints, in the neck or elsewhere. The
streptococci of these secondary foci may take on new
virulence and specific pathogenicity, from the same
causes which induced like changes in the pathogenic
bacteria of the primary focus.

RHEUMATIC ENDOCARDITIS, MYOCARDITIS AND PERICARDITIS

Endocarditis

We have noted the fact that certain strains of the
streptococcus rheumaticus have a greater affinity for
the endocardium than others. Endocarditis of the rheumatic type may be the only recognizable clinical entity,
especially in children, and may be so mild that it escapes

notice. Later a valvular scar defect may be manifest.
In rheumatic fever endocarditis occurs most frequently
in children. After twenty years it occurs less frequently

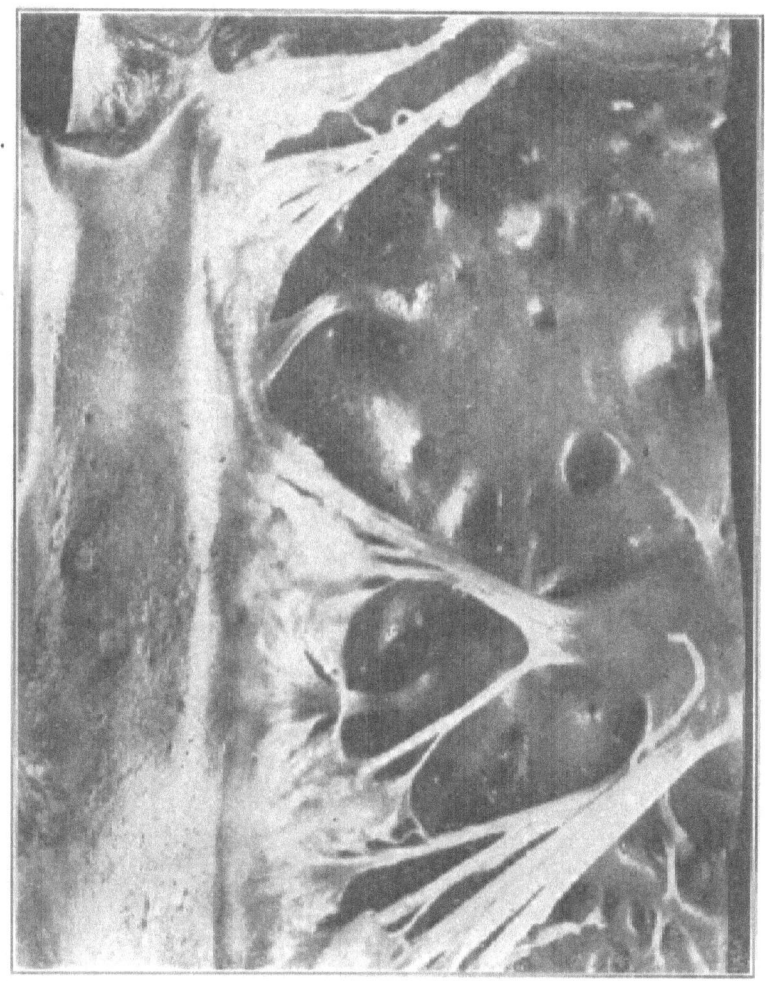

Fig. 8.—Subendothelial, Nodular, Valvular and Mural Endocarditis
of Dog Following Injection of "Streptococcus Rheumaticus."

during the first attack. The incidence of endocarditis
increases with the number of attacks, and always in
larger percentage in children.

As stated the virulence of the streptococcus rheumaticus is low, compared with other pathogenic strains of streptococci. Although this relatively low virulence may vary in degree and may become high, the morbid changes in joints and muscles consist at most of hyperemia and edematous swelling of the infected tissues. The changes in the endocardium are also characteristic of the usually mild virulence of the infectious bacteria as evinced by the mild tissue reaction in the form of small warty nodes of the endocardium and valve segments. Rarely is the endocarditis so severe as to be called ulcerative or malignant. When that condition occurs a change in type or in specific pathogenicity of the invading streptococci has probably occurred. Although rheumatic valvulitis is usually mild and is of itself rarely dangerous, the secondary sclerotic changes and retraction of the segments is an irremediable and harmful sequel.

Myocarditis

Myocarditis is undoubtedly a common incident in rheumatic fever only recognized clinically when marked cardiac incompetency occurs with or without dilatation. Mild myocarditis alone due to infection with streptococci which have a pathogenic affinity for muscular tissue undoubtedly occurs from chronic infectious foci. The mild reaction excited by the streptococci of low virulency in the walls of the heart is naturally in the form of proliferative interstitial tissue changes.

Pericarditis

Pericarditis may occur alone, in association with endocarditis, and may be involved in pancarditis in the course of rheumatic fever. It may occur as a simple fibrinous or serofibrinous type. Occasionally purulent pericarditis may occur with rheumatic fever in children. Pus in the pericardium or in a joint would indicate a coincident infection with pyogenic bacteria or a change in pathogenicity of the infectious agent, for the streptococcus rheumaticus. does not cause suppuration. In rheumatic fibrinous and serofibrinous pericarditis, the prognosis is good for recovery, but adhesions of the pericardial layers is a common sequel which later may cause nutritional disturbance of the heart muscle.

CHOREA

Acute chorea is an infectious disease. Its casual relation with rheumatic fever and the frequency of endocarditis of the simple rheumatic type in chorea indicate the infectious character and a common bacterial cause. The incidence of the disease is much the same as rheumatism. The first attack occurs most frequently in children between the ages of five and fifteen years. Seasonal incidence is the same as rheumatism. An attack of chorea may precede, occur with or follow an attack of rheumatic fever. Recurrent attacks usually occur. Pericarditis may occur. Recovery is the rule. The nervous phenomena, ataxic movements, muscular weakness, mental disturbances, mutism, etc., may occur by hematogenous infection, with a type of the strepto-

coccus rheumaticus which has a specific elective affinity
for the brain. Multiple cerebral bacterial embolism due
to a type of streptococcus of low virulence would cause
little anatomical disturbance, but could be provocative
of all the motor and sensory phenomena of the disease.
Indeed, gross embolism of the smaller cerebral vessels
has been found and has been the source of the etiologic
embolic theory. Simple verrucose endocarditis resem-
bling simple rheumatic endocarditis is the most common
morbid anatomical change in chorea. The cerebral
embolism theory is related to the associated endocarditis, with alleged detachment of small emboli composed
of fibrin, blood cells, etc. During life one may not study
the tissues of the brain as in other hematogenous infections of muscles, joints, lymph glands, etc. The
discovery of bacterial emboli in other infected tissues
of rheumatic fever, and the recognition of very slight resulting tissue reaction, is presumptive evidence that bacterial cerebral embolism may be the cause of chorea.
Rothstein and others have isolated strains of streptococci post mortem from the meninges of choreic individuals. Animal experimentation with specific strains
of the streptococcus isolated in rheumatic fever associated with chorea has been followed by joint infection
and characteristic symptoms of chorea in the inoculated
animals.

ACUTE SYSTEMIC GONOCOCCUS INFECTION

Gonococcemia may result from a local infection
of the prostate, seminal vesicles, joints and tendon
sheaths, from infected thrombi of the veins contigu-

ous to local gonococcus infection and also from infected thrombi of the venous sinuses of the uterus in the puerperium. Gonococcemia is a very serious condition, usually fatal when the cause of malignant endocarditis and childbed fever. Like other bacteria the gonococcus varies in degrees of virulence, and if mild the patient may recover from a gonococcemia even though the condition is associated with endocarditis, puerperal fever or suppurative arthritis. Thayer (57) has reported the recovery of two cases of gonococcus endocarditis. I have seen two patients recover who had suppurating multiple arthritis with gonococcemia. All of the suppurating joints were opened and drained, which doubtless aided recovery. The removal of the focal cause in all systemic gonorrheal infection may aid in overcoming the general disease.

Gonococcus Arthritis

Arthritis is the most frequent systemic expression of gonococcus focal infection. When monarticular the knee joint is most frequently involved. Males suffer in the proportion of twelve to one or two of females. It usually occurs during an acute gonorrhea, but may occur after the subsidence of an acute attack or from a long existing focal infection of the genito-urinary organs. For some reason the latent bacteria may take on new virulence and cause the late systemic manifestation. In women the focal lesion may be difficult to locate.

Anatomically it occurs as a synovitis, and periarthritis, with bursitis and tenovaginitis. The synovial joint effusion is usually serofibrinous and occasionally purulent. Purulent bursitis and tenovaginitis are more frequent. Periarthritis of the wrist with suppuration extending along the sheaths of tendons of the hands may occur. Periostitis of the os calcis with resulting exostosis and marked tenderness of the heel is a remarkable condition due to the gonococcus.

The gonococcus is present in the infected tissues and in the exudate of the joints, bursae and tendon sheaths from which with proper technic it may be recovered in pure culture. In chronic conditions the infection may be mixed with streptococci and staphylococci.

It is a most damaging and seriously disabling disease.

When the exudate is purulent, early operative relief may save the joint and tendon sheaths and preserve function. In non-purulent conditions the tendency is to a long obstinate course with resulting damage to the blood vessels of the infected tissues. This results in local malnutrition with the attendant metabolic changes in the joint and tendons with resulting deformity and loss of function.

Gonococcus arthritis is often mistaken for rheumatism. Unlike rheumatism it more frequently attacks tendon sheaths and the exudate is sometimes purulent. It may involve the intervertebral, temporomaxillary, sternoclavicular and sacro-iliac joints while rheumatism rarely does so. Both may be polyarticular. Gonorrheal arthritis is often very painful in undue proportion to the apparent local infection. As a rule the fever is not high. The ordinary antirheumatic drugs do not alter the clinical course. In many instances the removal of the infectious focus is followed by quick relief of the systemic disease.

MALIGNANT ENDOCARDITIS

Malignant or ulcerative endocarditis, so called because of the tendency to local tissue destruction and the high mortality which it causes, may be acute or chronic. It is always a secondary disease. It may be a local complication of a systemic disease like pneumonia, typhoid fever, epidemic cerebrospinal meningitis and rarely of rheumatic fever, or it may arise from a focal infection anywhere in the body due to the gonococcus, streptococcus, staphylococcus and less frequently to other infectious bacteria. There is always an associated bacteriemia. The bacteria which are most frequently found in the infected heart tissues, vegetations and contained thrombi, in the blood stream by cultures, are streptococci, pneumococci, gonococci and staphylococci. Streptococci are the most frequent cause and reach the blood stream and heart from septic wounds, the septic puerperal uterus, and other streptococcus foci about the head and elsewhere. While the streptococcus pyogenes is the strain which causes most of the acute types arising from acute infectious foci, the streptococcus viridans may also cause the acute type, but usually is the cause of chronic malignant endocarditis.

Bacteriemia associated with the general diseases named or due to a focal infection may not involve the heart. The normal endocardium is apparently resistant while old sclerotic processes of the valves and congenital deformities of the heart and proximal vessels predispose to malignant endocarditis. Hence malignant endocarditis most often occurs in individuals suffering from chronic valvular disease and chronic cardiomyopathy.

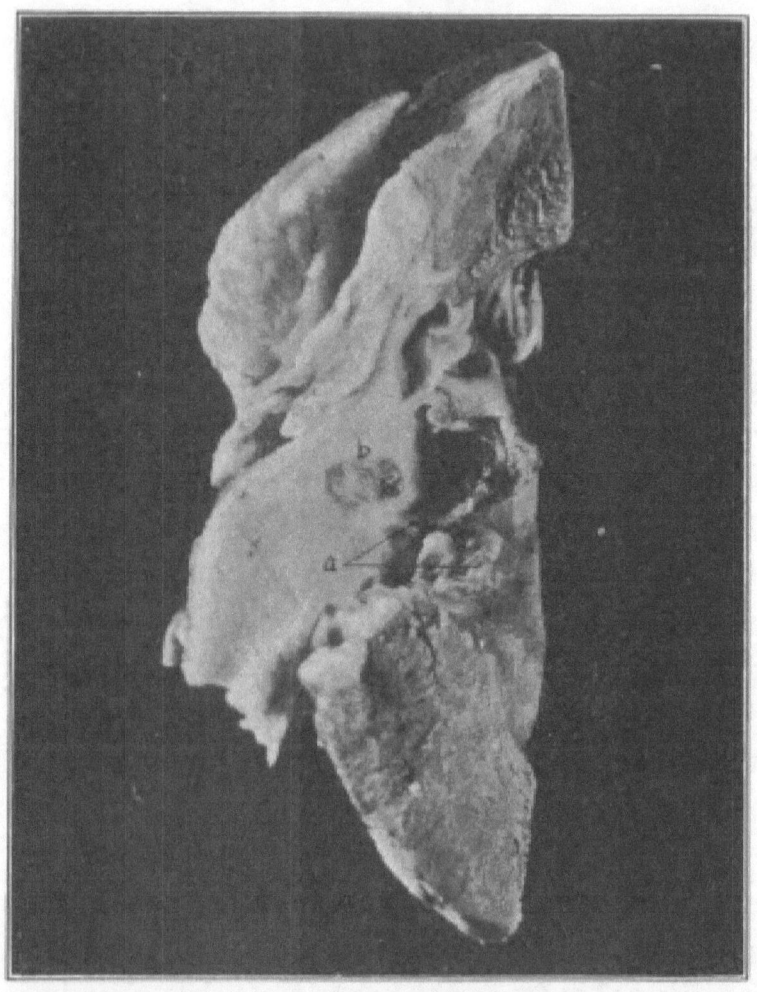

Fig. 9.—Vegetative and Ulcerative Endocarditis of Aortic Valves and Aorta of Dog Following Injection of Streptococcus Viridans from Chronic Vegetative Endocarditis of Man.

The morbid anatomy is essentially the same in all bacterial types of the acute form. Usually vegetations are present, often massive, especially when due to the pneumococcus, and streptococcus viridans. Occasionally the vegetations are not large while necrotic destructive lesions are dominant in very virulent infections and especially when staphylococci are the cause. From the cir-

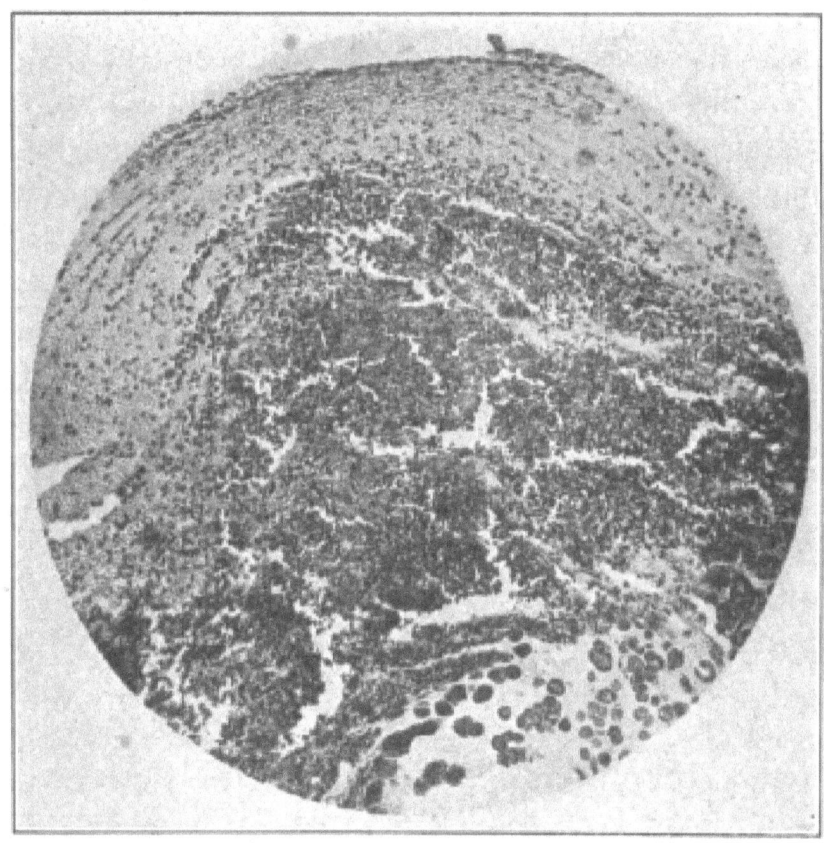

Fig. 10.—Section Through Vegetations on Mitral Valve Shown in Fig. 9. Note the dark areas consisting of clumps of streptococci.

culating blood thrombus formation occurs in the vegetations. Necrosis of endocardium, superficial and deep, with perforation of valves and other destructive lesions, may occur. The infectious bacteria are present in great number in the vegetations, thrombi and involved tissues.

. When malignant endocarditis occurs as a local complication of a general disease like pneumonia, rheumatic fever, cerebrospinal fever, or some other acute disease, it may not be recognized because the severe symptoms of the systemic disease may overshadow and mask the manifestations of the local condition. As a rule the other symptoms of the general disease are intensified with evidence of failing heart, leading to a rapid fatal issue. Frequently the severe endocarditis is first recognized at autopsy.

There are, however, special and characteristic symptoms which may lead to the recognition of the condition of the heart and especially if a bacteriemia is found by blood culture. Detached small particles of the vegetations and of thrombi carried in the blood stream may cause embolism in the various tissues and organs. Embolism may give rise to delirium, coma, paralysis, perisplenitis, with enlargement and tenderness of the spleen, varying degrees of hematuria, gangrene of distal tissues and petechiae, and at any point local abscesses may develop from the infected emboli. Mycotic aneurism may result. Embolism of lung followed by abscess may occur if the right heart is involved. Usually the local cardiac disease is manifested by endocardial murmurs, but may be absent. The septic type is marked by chills and an intermittent or remittent type of fever and severe sweats. A typhoid type is characterized by a more continued type of fever, delirium, coma and rapid course. In rare instances the clinical picture is that of cerebrospinal meningitis. The diagnosis may be difficult, but is greatly aided by blood culture.

Malignant endocarditis usually terminates fatally, but recovery has been noted by Herrick (21) and others In coroner's autopsy cases E. R. LeCount has recognized six or more instances of healed scars of ulcerative endocarditis.

ACUTE NEPHRITIS

The type of acute infectious nephritis which usually rises from a focal infection is embolic because the mode

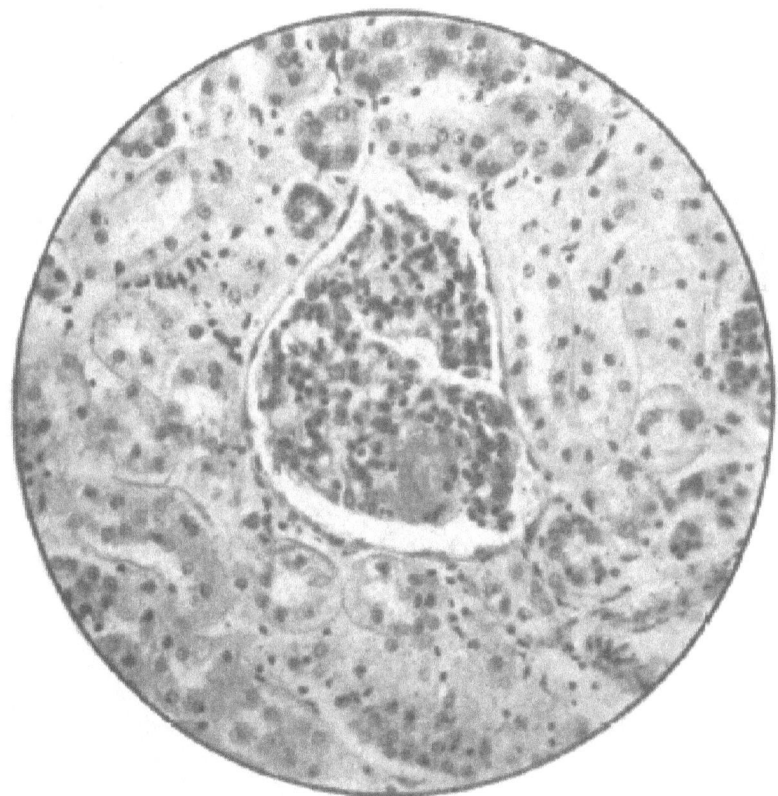

Fig. 11.—A Glomerulus Containing a Hyaline Thrombus. From a rabbit dying 7 days after inoculation. X 275 (after LeCount and Jackson, Jour. Inf. Dis.).

of infection is hematogenous. It is, therefore, primarily a glomerulonephritis. If the dose of infectious bacteria

reaching the kidney is large enough, the nephritis may
be diffuse. Usually the condition is expressed clinically
by bloody urine of varying degree, microscopic blood
is present with albuminuria and casts of various

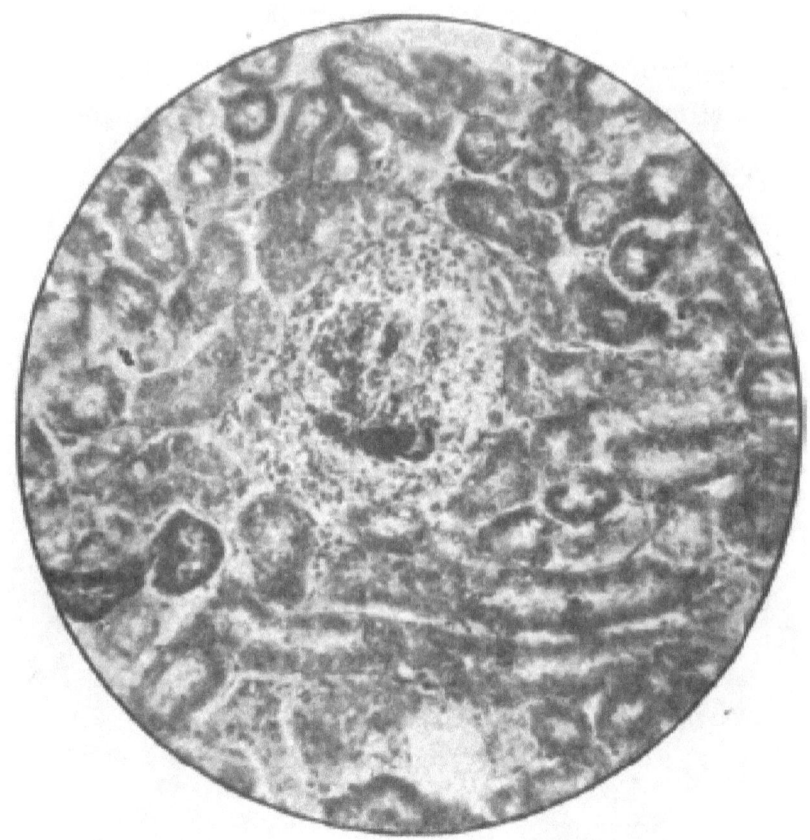

Fig. 12.—Masses of Fibrin in a Glomerulus. From rabbit dying 7 days
after injection. X 200 (after LeCount and Jackson, Jour. Inf. Dis.).

types. The urine is lessened in quantity in twenty-
four hours, soon a secondary anemia develops and
often within a short period a soft edema. Varying degrees of this type of nephritis occur from focal infection. The most usual site of the focal infection which
causes the nephritis is the throat. In the milder types

of this form of nephritis apparent complete resolution occurs after the removal of the focus of infection. Billings (9) has reported clinical observations on the relation of focal infection to glomerulonephritis and the

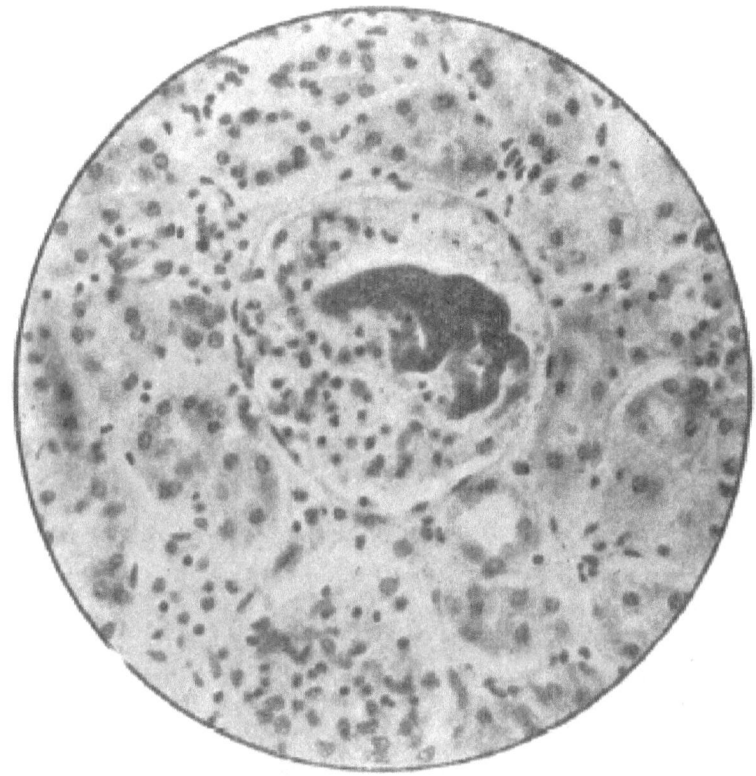

Fig. 13.—A Glomerulus in Which Are Masses of Cocci Filling a Group of Capillaries. From a rabbit dying 9 days after inoculation. X 325 (after LeCount and Jackson, Jour. Inf. Dis.).

apparent resolution of the infection of the kidneys by eradication of the focus. LeCount and Jackson (35) have shown the renal changes in rabbits inoculated with streptococci. Of these animals six were inoculated with strains of streptococci isolated from patients with epidemic septic angina. The kidney lesions were primarily of the vascular structures, glomeruli, intertubular vessels and arcuate and interlobar veins. They noted a pronounced perivascular exudate consisting chiefly of lymphocytes and plasma cells. The tendency to repair in the acute glomerular lesion, noted by LeCount and Jackson, is very important when compared with the tendency to recovery of clinical glomerulonephritis of man, when the chief etiologic factor is removed.

ACUTE APPENDICITIS

Acute appendicitis due to focal infection located in the throat and nose and sometimes in the jaws has been noted by a great number of clinical observers, notably among the French. Kretz (25) has shown the frequent infection of the cervical lymph nodes with streptococci. When the cause of the lymphogenous infection is acute Kretz believes that the bacteria filtrate rapidly through the lymph nodes, with resulting severe bacteriemia. In less severe types of focal infection of the head and in adults especially, the virulence and degree of bacteriemia is usually less. In these conditions, local or general systemic infection may follow in the form of acute multiple arthritis (rheumatism), endocarditis, pericarditis, osteomyelitis, nephritis, appendicitis, cholecystitis and even streptococcus malignant endocarditis. He also believes that acute appendicitis and cholecystitis are hematogenous in origin and never primarily caused by infection within the lumen of the appendix and gall-bladder. Cannon (26) argues that appendicitis and cholecystitis are hematogenous infections, and may be of focal origin. He believes that typhoid cholecystitis occurs through the blood stream.

After animal experimentation and a study of the tissues and bacteria of appendicitis, Ghon and Namba

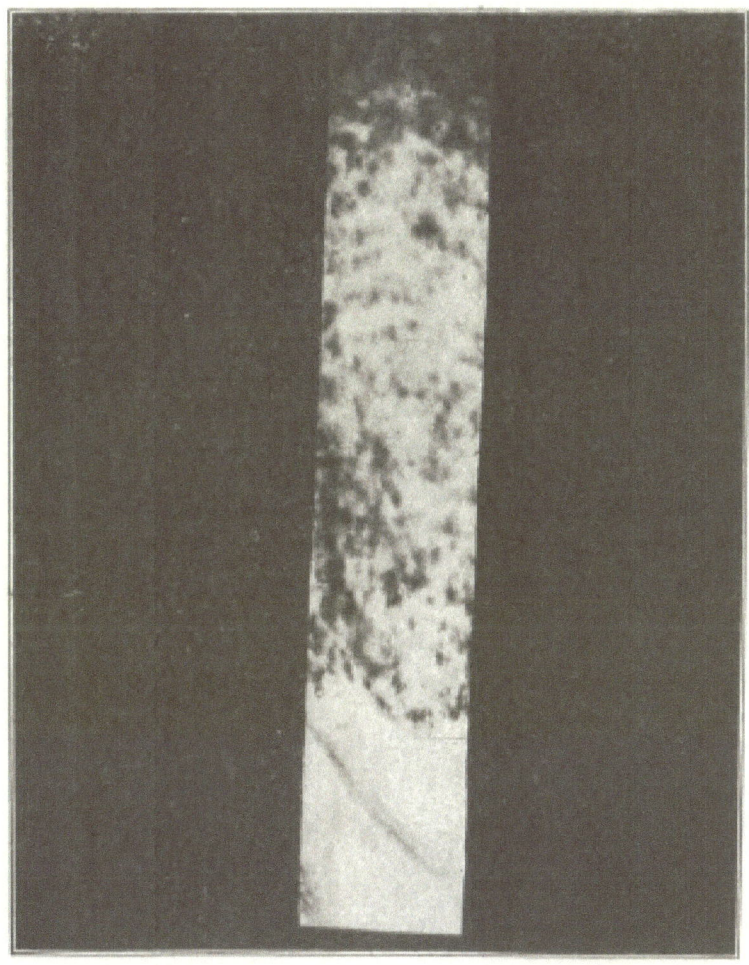

Fig 14.—Marked Hemorrhage of the Appendix 24 Hours After Injection of Streptococci from Tonsils in a Case of Human Appendicitis.

(27) conclude that if appendicitis occurs hematogenously it must be due to a specific strain of streptococci.

Adrian (28) has observed appendicitis as a focal infection of general disease. He apparently considers the bacteriemia of a focal infection a general disease.

Hence he cites clinical observation of angina, with appendicitis. He very fully reviews the literature quoting the opinion of many German, French and a few Amer-

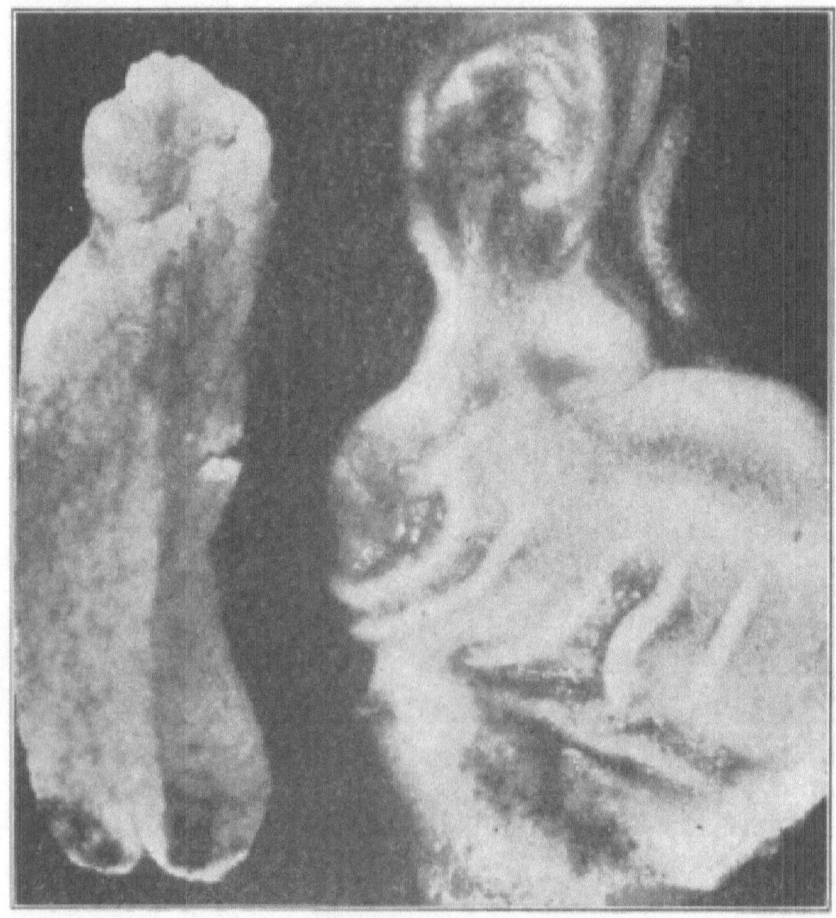

Fig. 15.—Hemorrhage and Localized Infection of Mucous Membrane of Duodenum and Tip of Appendix 48 Hours After Injection of Streptococcus from Human Appendicitis After Three Animal Passages.

ican clinicians upon the relation of angina to appendicitis and rheumatism. The histologic lymphoid structure of the tonsils and appendix is compared and the similarity of tissue is given as a reason for the etiological relation of the angina to appendicitis. The term "anginal appendicitis" has been coined to express this relation.

The confirmatory investigations of Rosenow (8) have shown the occurrence of acute appendicitis from strains

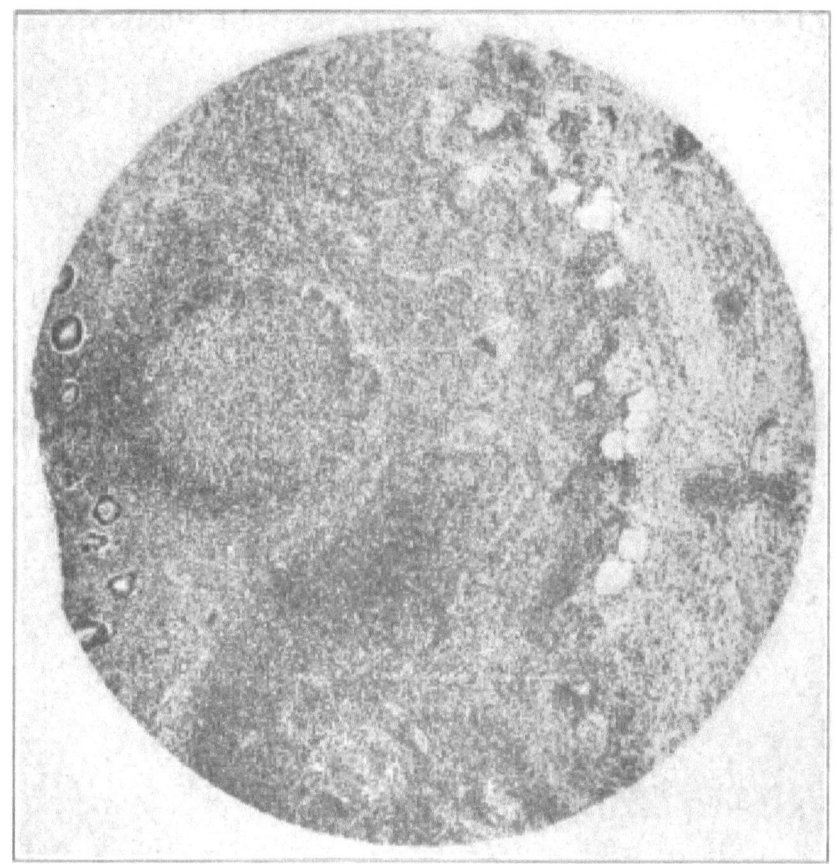

Fig. 16.—Human Appendicitis 12 Hours After Onset in Young Man. Note the necrosis and infiltration of lymph follicles.

of streptococci, colon bacilli and other organisms which have attained elective affinity for the tissues of the appendix. This elective tissue affinity has been acquired by these microörganisms in the tissues of the appendix during an attack, for when they are isolated from the

infected tissues of the appendix and nascent cultures
are injected intravenously into animals, acute appendicitis occurs in the great majority of the inoculated
animals. The same affinity for tissues of the appendix
can be induced to appear in strains through variations
in culture methods and serial animal inoculation.

Fig. 17.—Diplococci in Peritoneal Coat of Appendix Shown in Fig. 16.

The invading organisms reaching the tissues of the
appendix hematogenously cause small hemorrhages in
the walls of the organ and if this invasion is great
enough the reaction of the tissues to the invading
organisms causes a positive chemotaxis with invasion
of leukocytes and plasma cells and consequent tumefac-
tion of the tissues and obstruction of the canal of the
appendix. With obstruction there occurs a condition
which invites the rapid increase in the numerous saprophytic anaerobes and other bacteria usually present in

the bowel and appendix with resulting increase of morbid tissue change, varying in degree from edema to necrosis and gangrene. Until these investigations of Rosenow, the presence of colon bacteria and of various

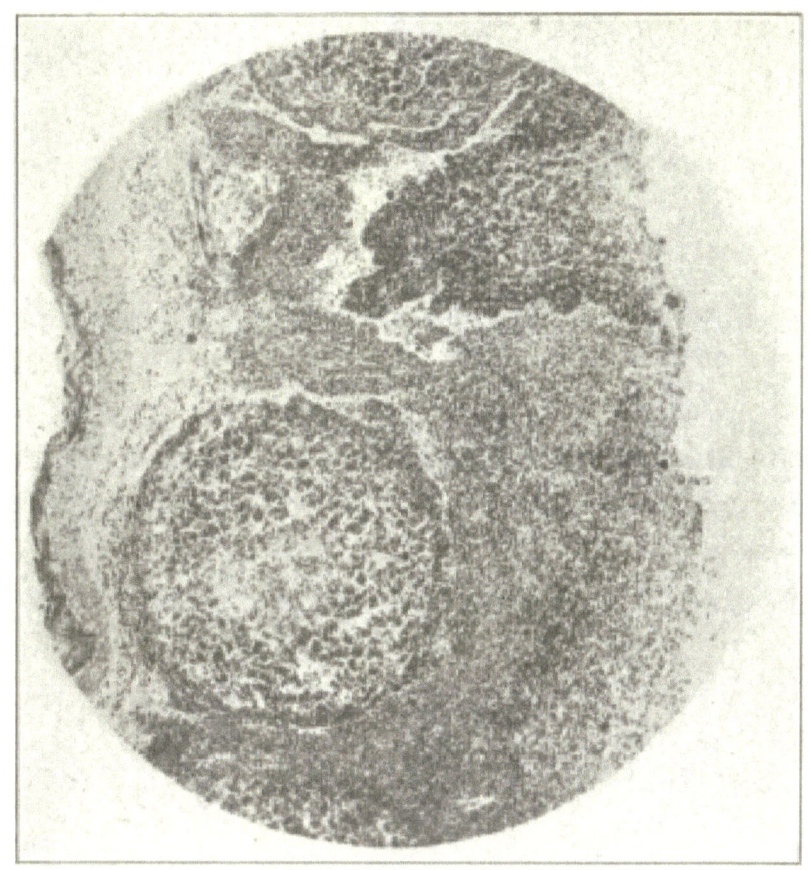

Fig. 18.—Hemorrhage Necrosis and Leukocytic Infiltration 20 Hours After Injection of Streptococcus from Appendix in Human Appendicitis After One Animal Passage.

other saprophytic organisms in the tissues of the normal as well as the infected appendix, has led to the belief that acute appendicitis has been excited by an infection within the bowel by the various saprophytic organisms usually found there. This secondary invasion of anae-

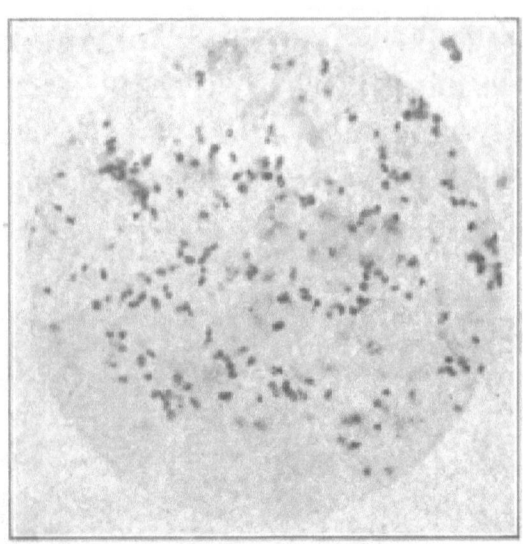

Fig. 19.—Streptococci in Lymph Follicle Shown in Fig. 18 of Appendix 20 Hours After Injection of Streptococci.

robes and other bacteria often found in the tissues closely related to the intestinal tract have been described as the primary causes of appendicitis by Heyde (29), Aschoff (30) and others. The argument from

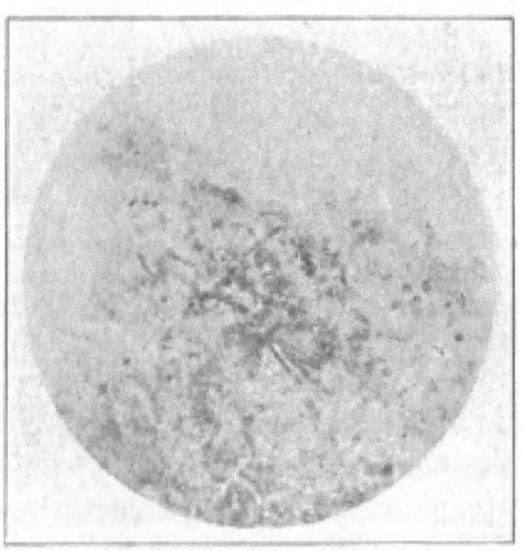

Fig. 20.—Streptococci and Fusiform Bacilli in Human Gangrenous Appendicitis Following Vincent's Angina.

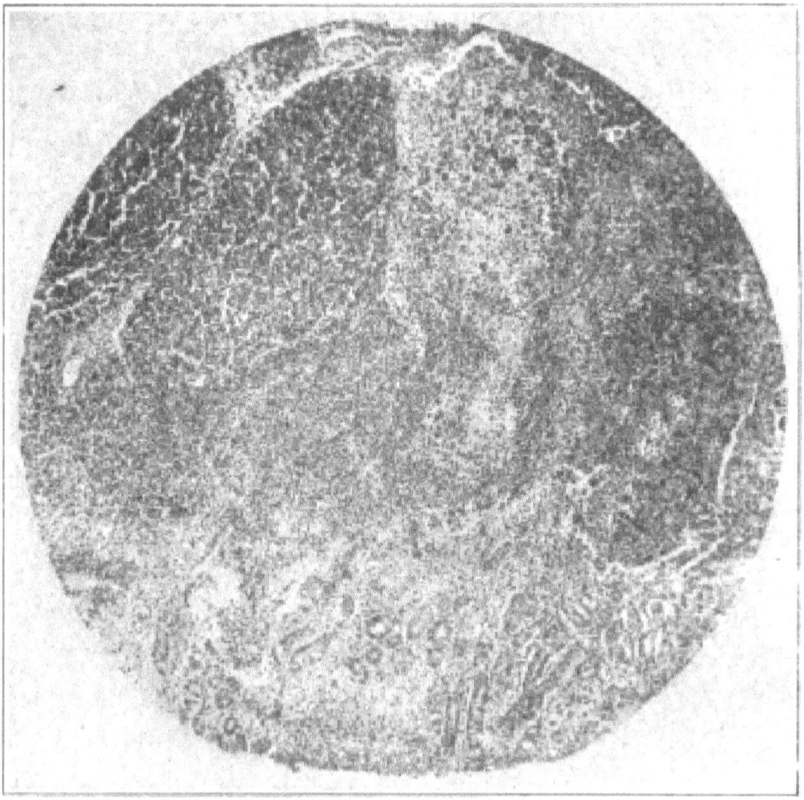

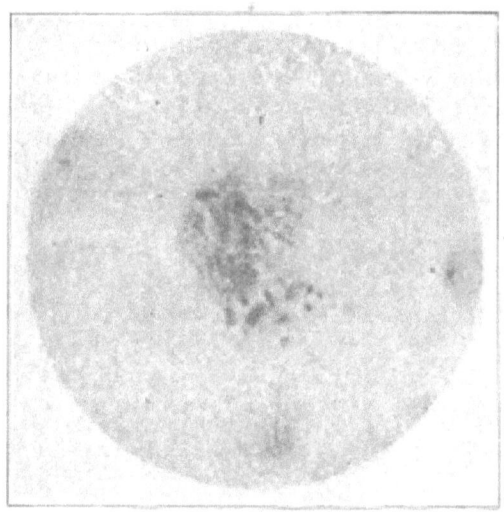

Fig. 21.—Hemorrhage, Necrosis and Leukocytic Infiltration of Appendix 24 Hours After Injection of Mixed Culture of Fusiform Bacilli and Streptococci from Human Appendix Shown in Fig. 20.

Fig. 22.—Streptococci and Fusiform Bacilli of Appendix of Rabbit Shown in Fig. 21 24 Hours After Intravenous Injection.

this point of view is that these facultative bacteria invade the tissues from the lumen of the bowel, when the resistance of the body tissues is low, and especially when the lumen of the appendix is partly or wholly closed by fecal concretions, kinks of the organ or from other causes. The more reasonable relation of these bacteria

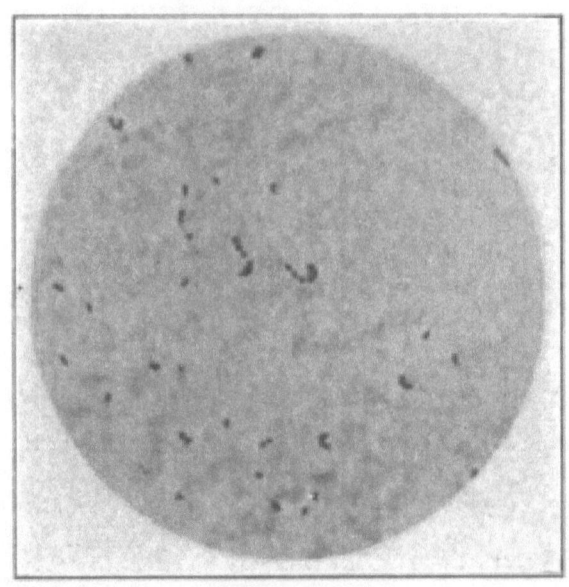

Fig. 23.—Photomicrograph of 24 Hour Culture in Ascites-Dextrose-Broth of a Streptococcus Isolated from a Gall-bladder in Human Cholecystitis. The morphology, size and grouping are quite typical of strains from cholecystitis. Gram stain.

to the disease is that of a mixed infection, secondary to the primary hematogenous invasion usually by streptococci.

How much the lessened resistance of the tissues of the appendix due to the presence of fecal stones and other foreign bodies or to kinking of the organ may have to do in attracting the streptococci in the blood stream to the appendix, needs further investigation.

CHOLECYSTITIS

Cholecystitis is unquestionably due at times to hematogenous infection with strains of streptococci and pos-

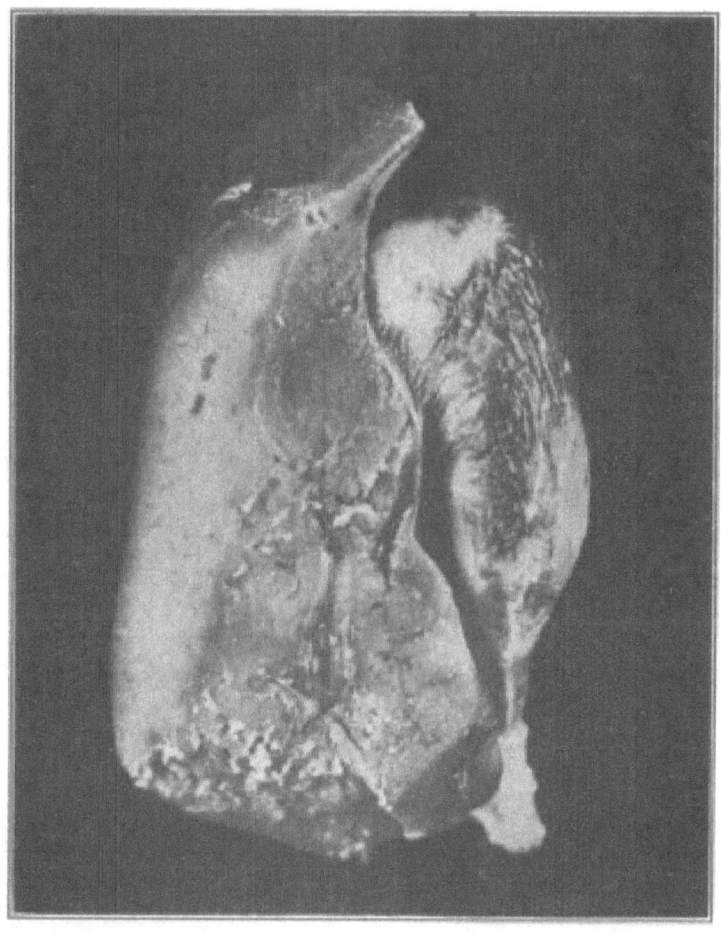

Fig. 24.—Hemorrhagic Cholecystitis in Dog 48 Hours After Intravenous Injection of Streptococcus Shown in Fig. 23, from the Thickened and Infiltrated Wall of Human Gall-bladder Soon After Isolation.

sibly to other microörganisms. A patient in the Presbyterian Hospital who suffered from an attack of acute cholecystitis was operated and it was noted that in the fundus of the gall-bladder there was a small softened area which was excised. The gall-bladder also contained some small soft concretions of bile. From the softened

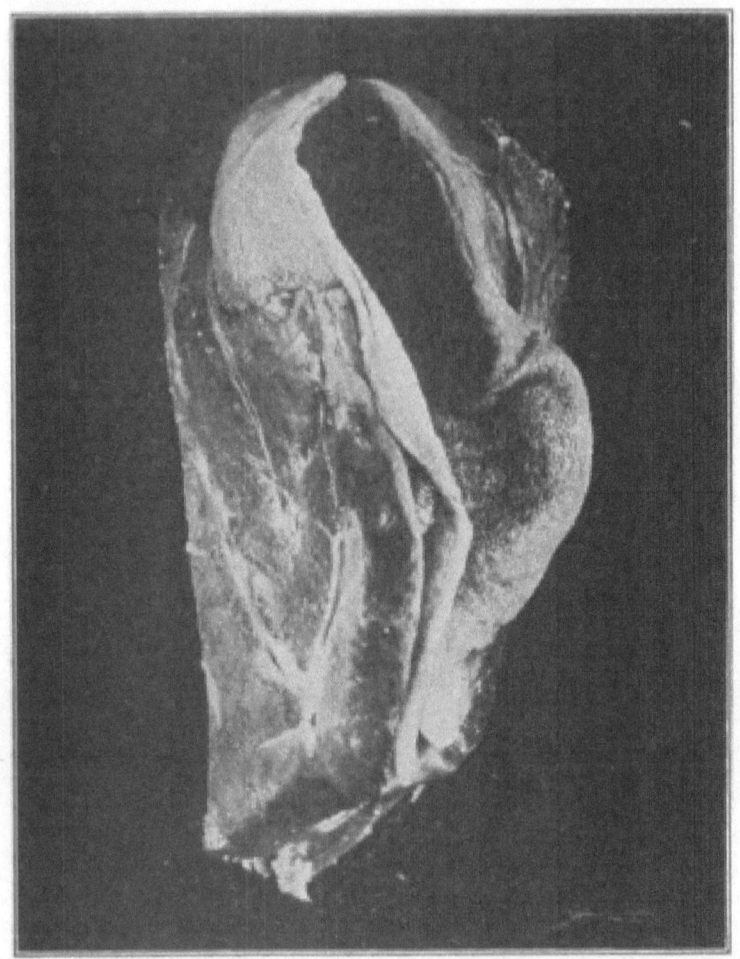

Fig. 25.—Marked Edema of Gall-bladder in Dog 24 Hours After Intravenous Injection of a Streptococcus from Duodenal Ulcer After One Animal Passage.

tissues of the gall-bladder Rosenow isolated a strain of streptococci which injected into animals produced cholecystitis. This patient suffered from tonsillitis and a short period before the onset of the attack of cholecys-

titis had suffered from an acute tonsillitis. Strains of
the streptococci isolated from the tonsil had a like affinity for the gall-bladder in intravenously inoculated
animals.

Rosenow has shown also that strains of the streptococci attain an affinity for the gall-bladder similar to

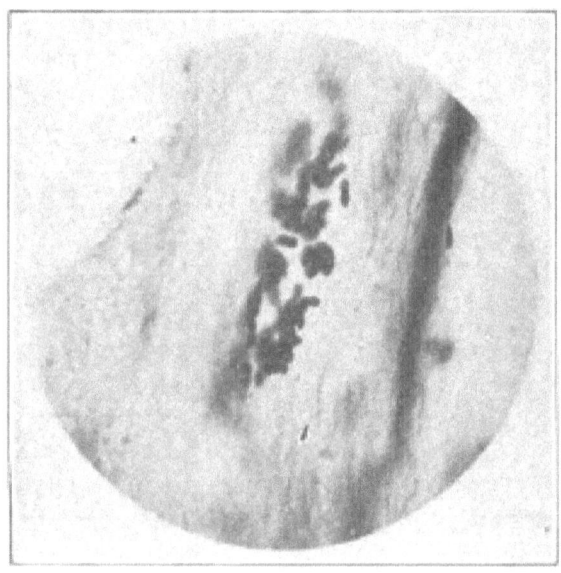

Fig. 26.—Streptococci in Lymph Space of Edematous Wall of Gall-
bladder Shown in Fig. 25. Gram-Weigert stain.

that attained for other tissues, and that this affinity may
be lost and regained by varying methods of culture and
by serial animal passage.

There can be no question that cholecystitis may occur
through hematogenous infection by typhoid bacilli and
probably by other pathogenic microörganisms, but the
more frequent presence of streptococci than the other
pathogenic bacteria in the center of gall-stones removed
from patients, as shown by Rosenow, is suggestive of

the more frequent occurrence of streptococcus cholecystitis.

ACUTE GASTRIC AND DUODENAL ULCER

Acute peptic, gastric and duodenal ulcer may be produced experimentally in animals by the intravenous

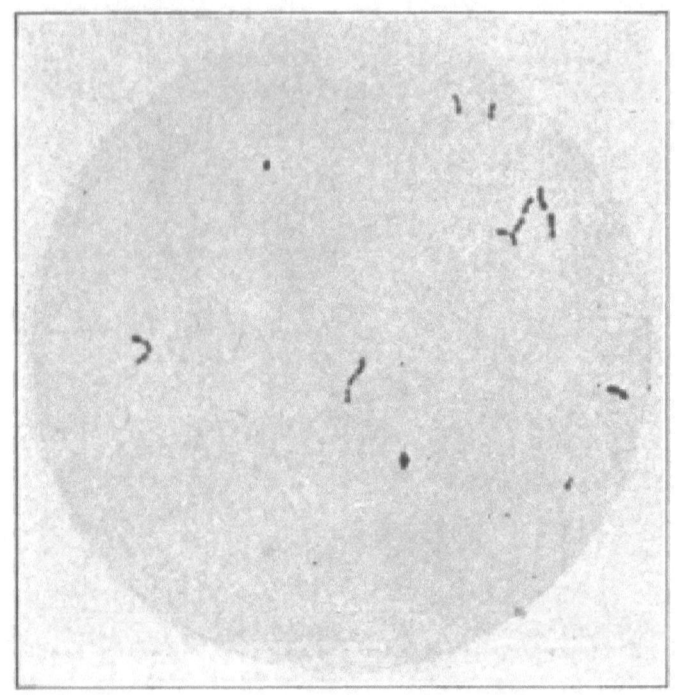

Fig. 27.—Photomicrograph of 24 Hour Ascites-Dextrose-Broth Culture of Streptococcus from Human Ulcer at the Time the Strain Proved to Have the Affinity for the Stomach When Intravenously Injected Into Animals. Grain stain.

injection of strains of streptococci which have an elective affinity for the stomach wall and Rosenow has isolated this strain from the base of the ulcer and tissue of the stomach wall of man. The strain, so isolated, proved to have an elective affinity for the stomach wall in animals intravenously inoculated. The mode of pro-

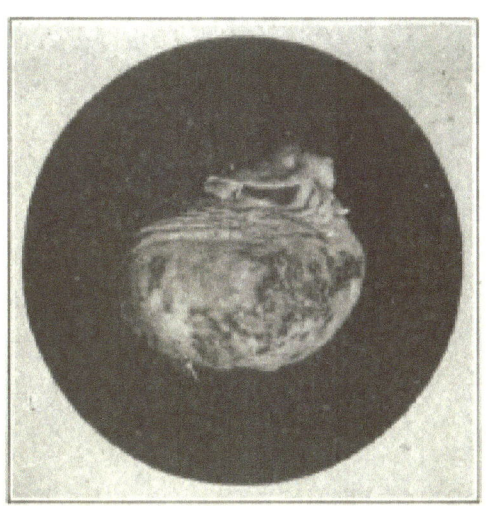

FIG. 28.—MARKED ULCERATION OF STOMACH IN GUINEA PIG 24 HOURS AFTER INTRAVENOUS INJECTION OF STREPTOCOCCUS FROM SUPPURATING FRONTAL SINUS OF MAN WITH STOMACH ULCER.

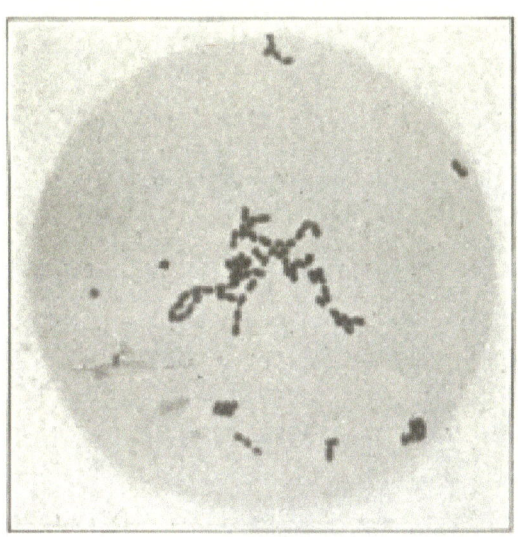

FIG. 29.—PHOTOMICROGRAPH 24 HOUR ASCITES-DEXTROSE-BROTH CULTURE OF A STREPTOCOCCUS FROM BLIND ABSCESS OF JAW IN MAN SUFFERING WITH CHRONIC ULCER OF STOMACH. This strain proved to have an affinity for the stomach when intravenously injected into animals. Gram stain.

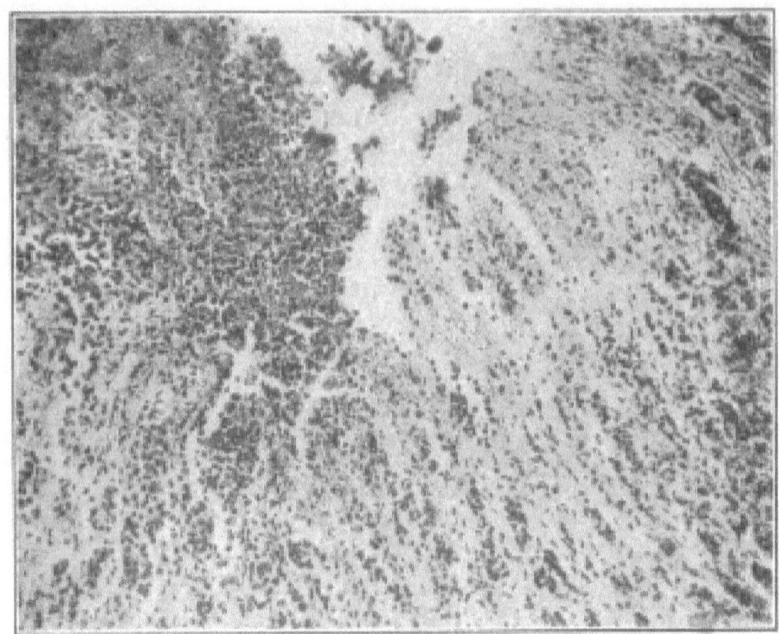

Fig. 30.—Ulcer of Stomach of Dog 5 Days After Intravenous Injection of Streptococcus from Human Ulcer.

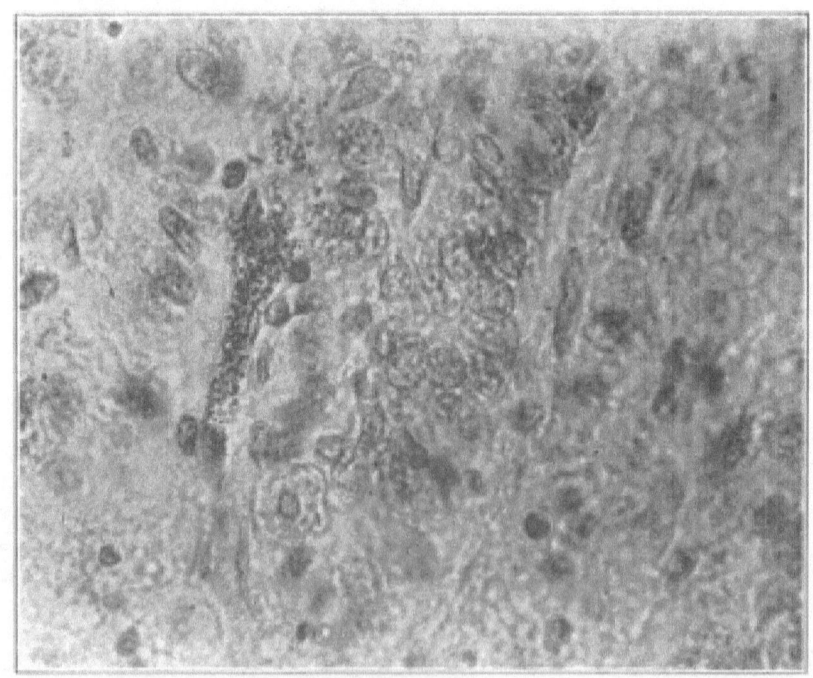

Fig. 31.—Capillary Filled with Diplococci in the Apex of the Ulcer Shown in Fig. 30.

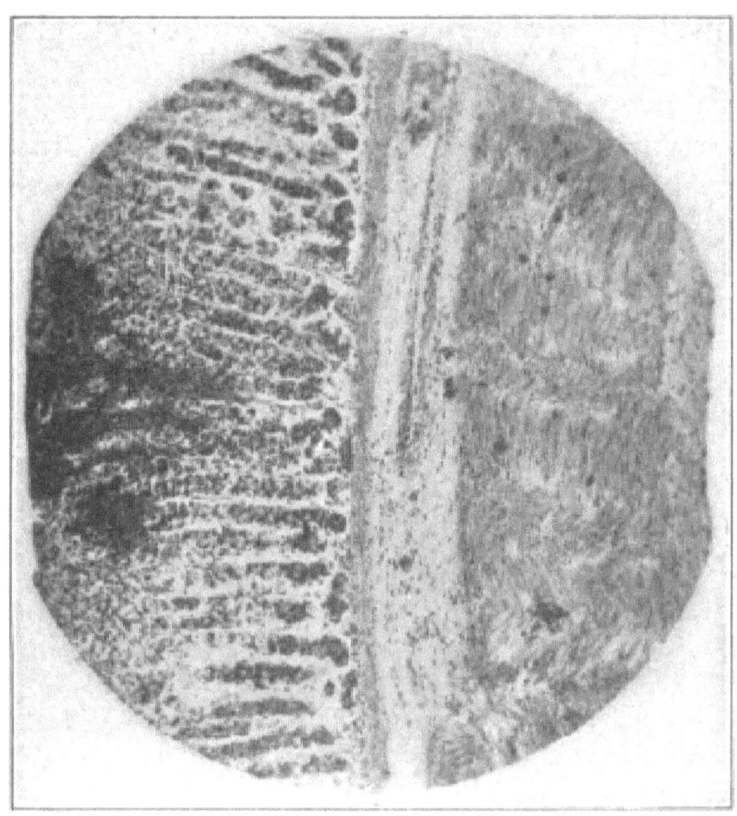

FIG. 32.—SECTION OF WALL OF STOMACH OF RABBIT SHOWING WEDGE-
SHAPED AREA OF INFILTRATION, HEMORRHAGE AND BEGINNING ULCERA-
TION 48 HOURS AFTER INTRAVENOUS INJECTION OF STREPTOCOCCI FROM
TONSIL OF PATIENT WITH HERPES ZOSTER AFTER ONE ANIMAL PASSAGE.

duction of the ulcer as noted   animals is a streptococcus embolic infection of the submucosa of the stomach with resulting small hemorrhages into the surrounding tissues.   In consequence of the hemorrhage and the

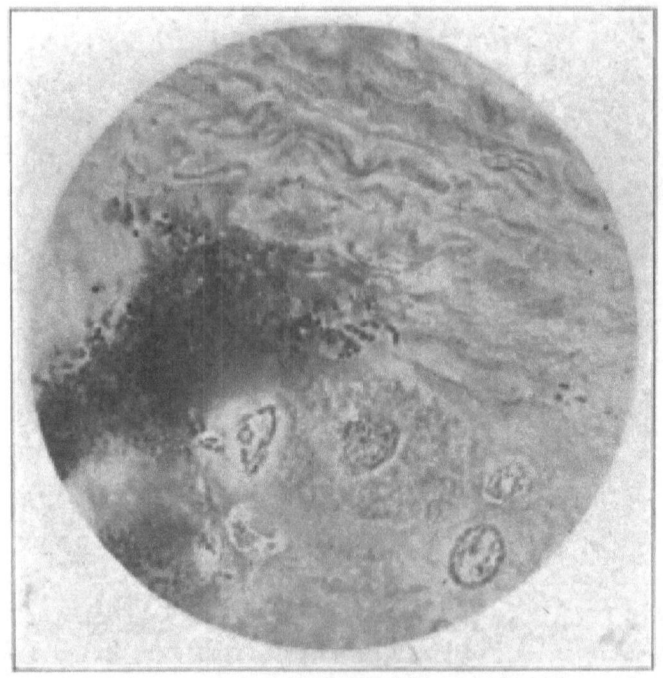

Fig. 33.—Streptococci at Apex of Wedge-Shaped Area Shown in Fig. 32.

presence of the infectious microörganisms in the surrounding tissues, anemic necrosis so weakens the over-
lying mucous membrane that it becomes digested by the
gastric juice.   If the necrosis involves a vessel of sufficient size, visible stomach hemorrhage may occur.   If
the infection and injury is not great, healing takes place.
If the infection is more virulent, chronic ulcer results.

ACUTE PANCREATITIS

Acute pancreatitis of serious degree always requires surgical interference. When it is of mild degree sur-

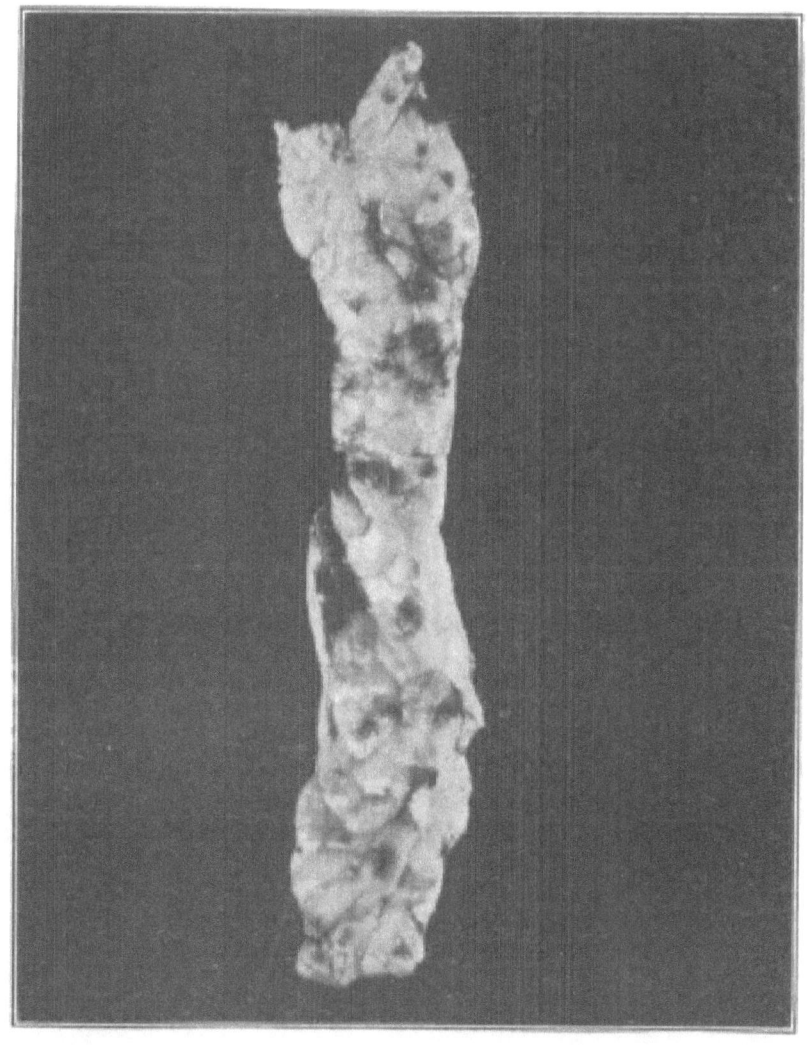

FIG. 34.—HEMORRHAGIC PANCREATITIS IN DOG 24 HOURS AFTER INJECTION OF STREPTOCOCCUS FROM STENO'S DUCT IN A CASE OF EPIDEMIC PAROTITIS.

gical interference is not usually required, but if it becomes a chronic condition degenerative changes may

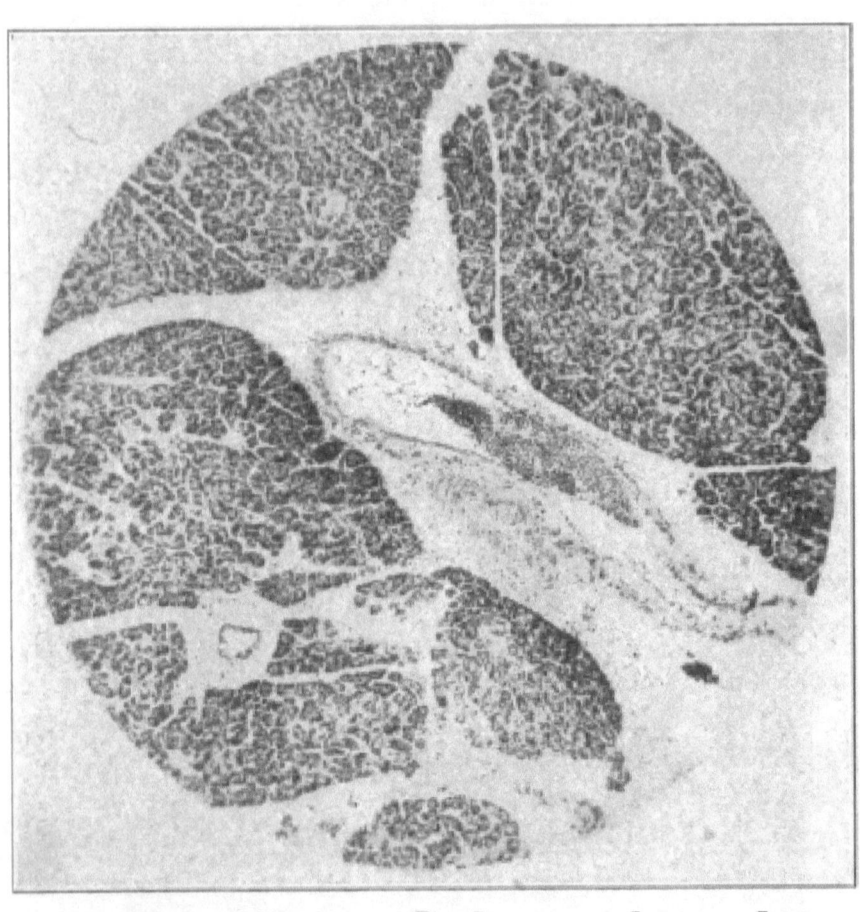

FIG. 35.—SECTION OF PANCREAS IN DOG SHOWING AN IRREGULAR STAINING OF PARENCHYMATOUS CELLS AND THROMBOSIS OF BLOOD VESSELS TWO WEEKS AFTER INTRAVENOUS INJECTION OF STREPTOCOCCI FROM RHEUMATISM.

lead to involvement of the islands of Langerhans with disturbed function and diabetes mellitus may result.

There is a relation more or less close between the strains of streptococci which have an elective tissue af-

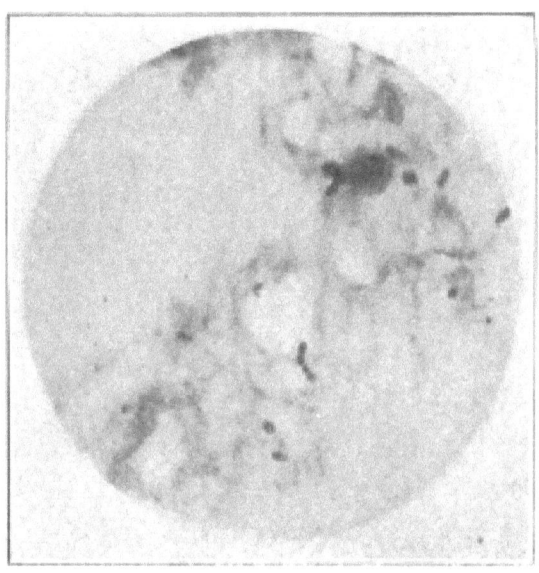

FIG. 36.—PHOTOMICROGRAPH SHOWING DIPLOCOCCI IN AREA OF ROUND CELL INFILTRATION NEAR A PARTIALLY THROMBOSED BLOOD VESSEL OF FIG. 35.

finity for the appendix, gall-bladder, stomach wall and pancreas and this has been beautifully and graphically shown in the table, which was presented in Lecture II.

ERYTHEMA NODOSUM

Erythema nodosum has been recognized as a condition which may occur with acute or subacute rheumatism or as a part of the syndrome described by Osler (17). The syndrome consists usually of polymorphic skin lesions, hyperemia, edema, hemorrhage, quite frequently associated with arthritis. At times there may

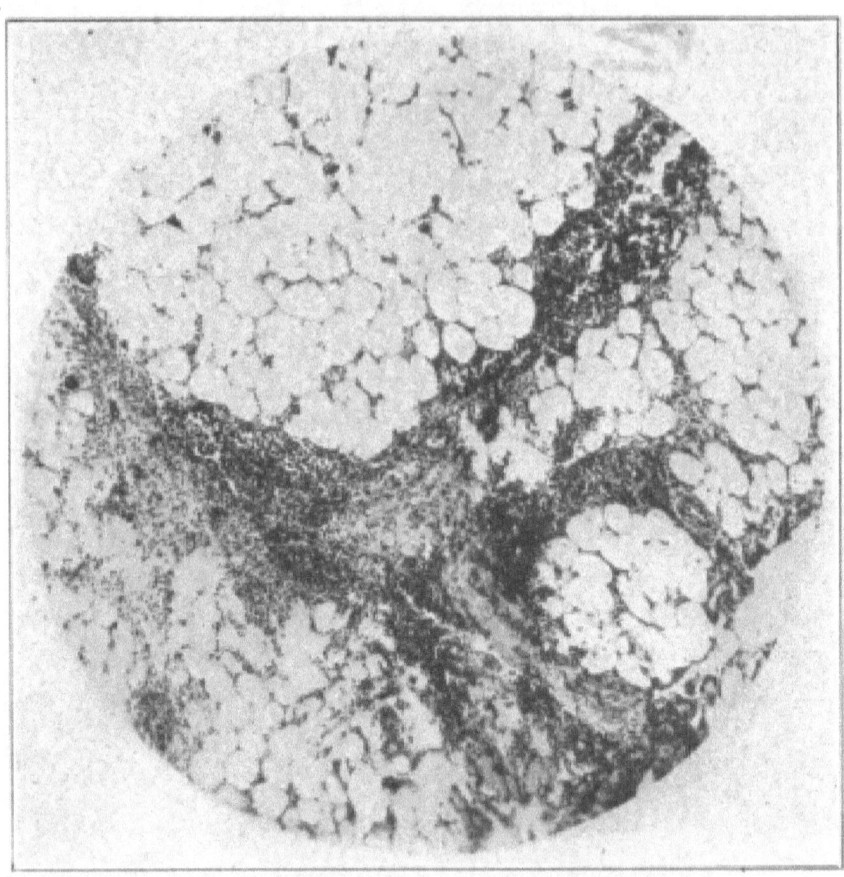

Fig. 37.—Subcutaneous Tissues from Erythema Nodosum in Man. Sections showing a leukocytic and round cell infiltration along tissue strands between the layers of fat.

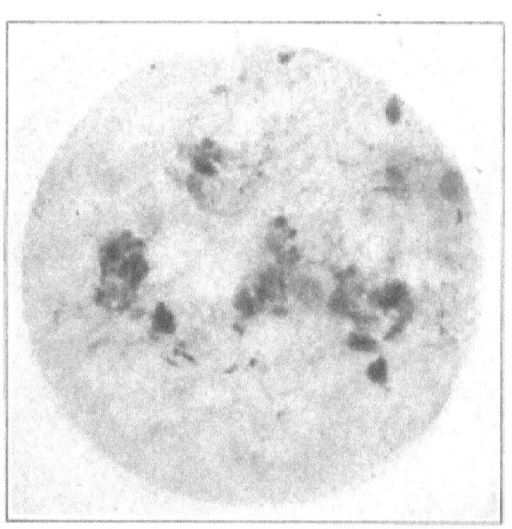

Fig. 38.—Subcutaneous Tissue from Erythema Nodosum in Man. Section showing red blood corpuscles, blood pigment, nuclei of disintegrated leukocytes and diplococci and diphtheroid bacilli.

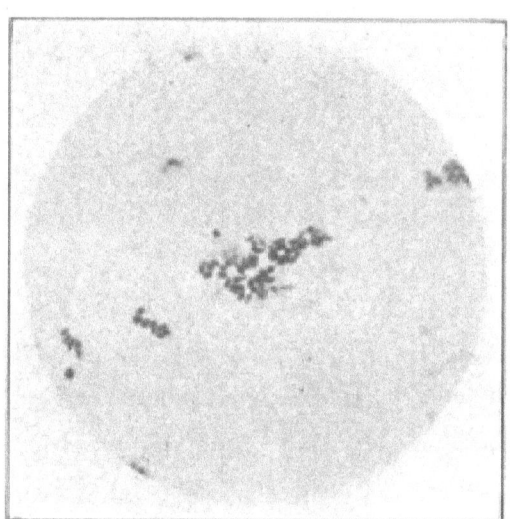

Fig. 39.—Smear from Single Colony in Ascites-Dextrose-Agar 72 Hours After Inoculation with the Emulsion of the Subcutaneous Node Showing Diphtheroid Bacilli in Fig. 38.

be visceral crises, especially gastro-intestinal, endocarditis, pericarditis, hematuria, nephritis, nodose erythema
and peliosis rheumatica. The present knowledge of
the infectious nature of rheumatism, of endocarditis,
pericarditis and nephritis, point to a probable focal infection as the cause of the syndrome, which has been

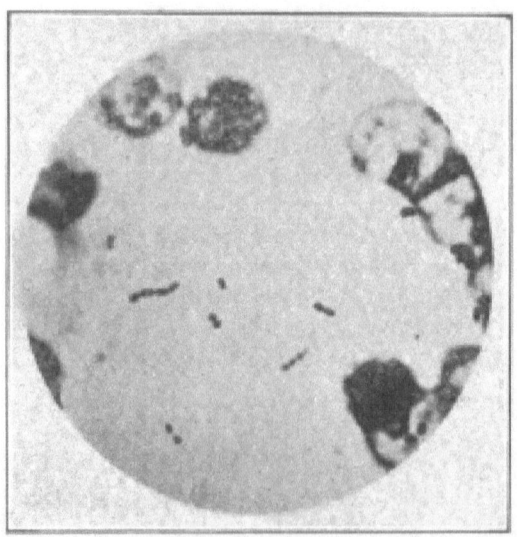

Fig. 40.—Smear from Blood of Guinea Pig Injected with Culture
Shown in Fig. 39 After One Animal Passage. Note the typical
diplococci in chains.

discussed by clinicians in the past, as infectious, toxic
or metabolic.

The discovery of bacteria belonging apparently
to the members of the streptococcus-pneumococcus
group in fresh tissues isolated from the nodes removed
surgically from patients and the production of erythema
nodosum in the skin of animals intravenously injected
with the cultures so obtained, has been demonstrated
many times by Rosenow.

The removal of the apparent focus of infection in

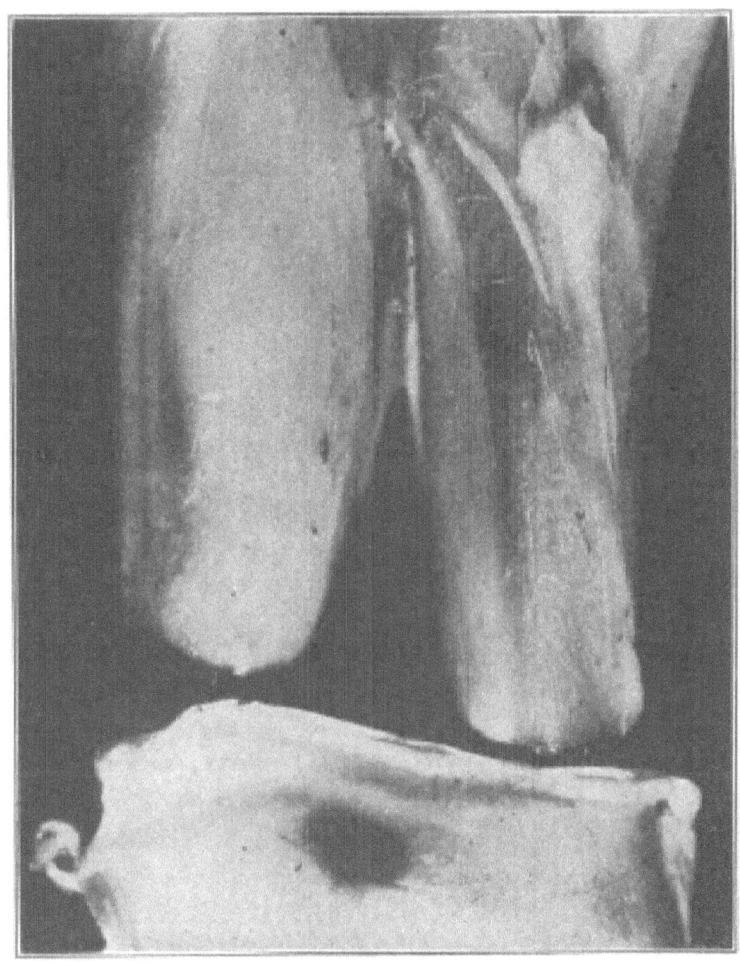

Fig. 41.—Photograph Showing Circumscribed Hemorrhages of the Skin and Symmetrical Hemorrhages of the Fascia of the Inner Aspect of the Legs of a Rabbit 48 Hours After an Intravenous Injection of Culture of Diphtheroid Bacteria Shown in Fig. 39, Obtained from an Erythematous Node in Man.

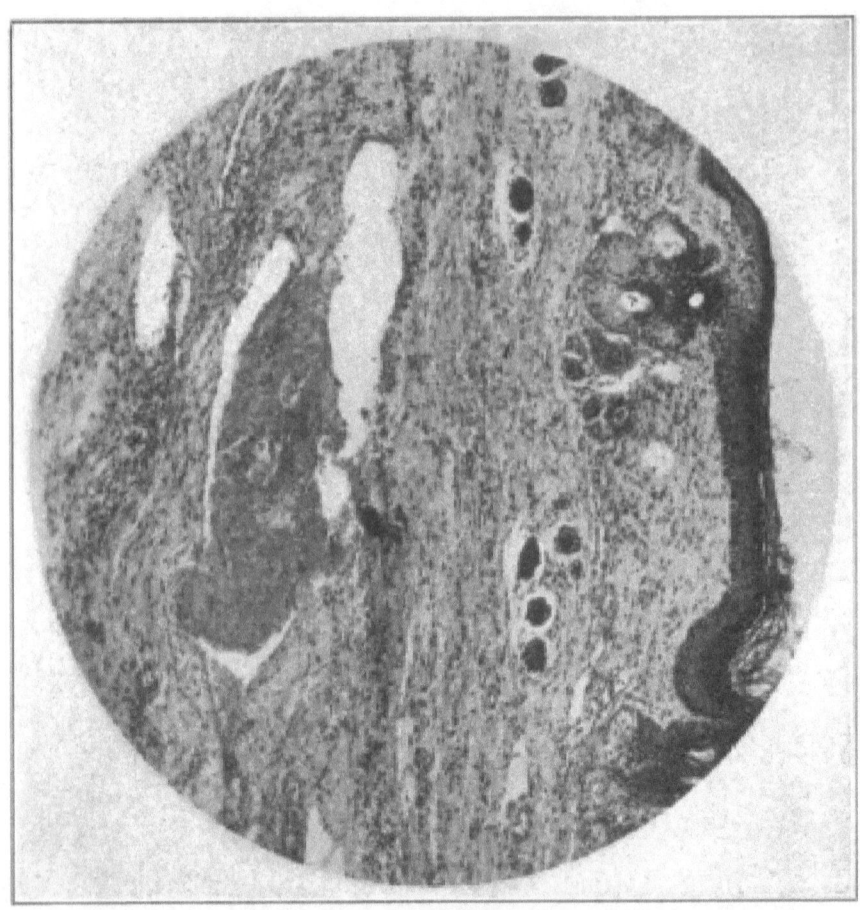

FIG. 42.—SECTION OF SKIN OF RABBIT SHOWING HEMORRHAGE AND LEU-
KOCYTIC AND ROUND CELL INFILTRATION OF SUBCUTANEOUS TISSUE 72
HOURS AFTER INTRAVENOUS INJECTION OF THE DIPHTHEROID BACILLI,
SHOWN IN FIG. 39. Note the complete absence of involvement of the
cutis and only slight infiltration of the corium.

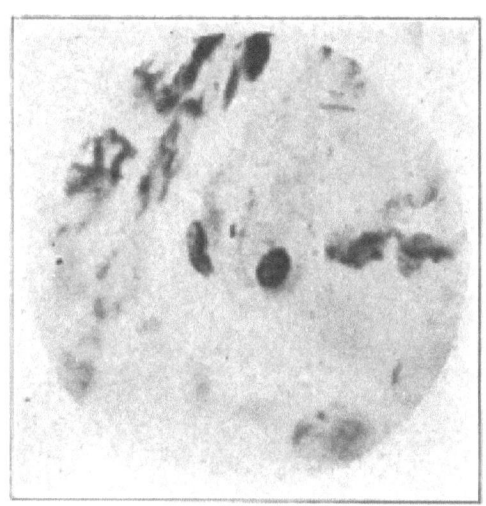

Fig. 43.—A Diplococcus in the Area of Infiltration Shown in Fig. 42.

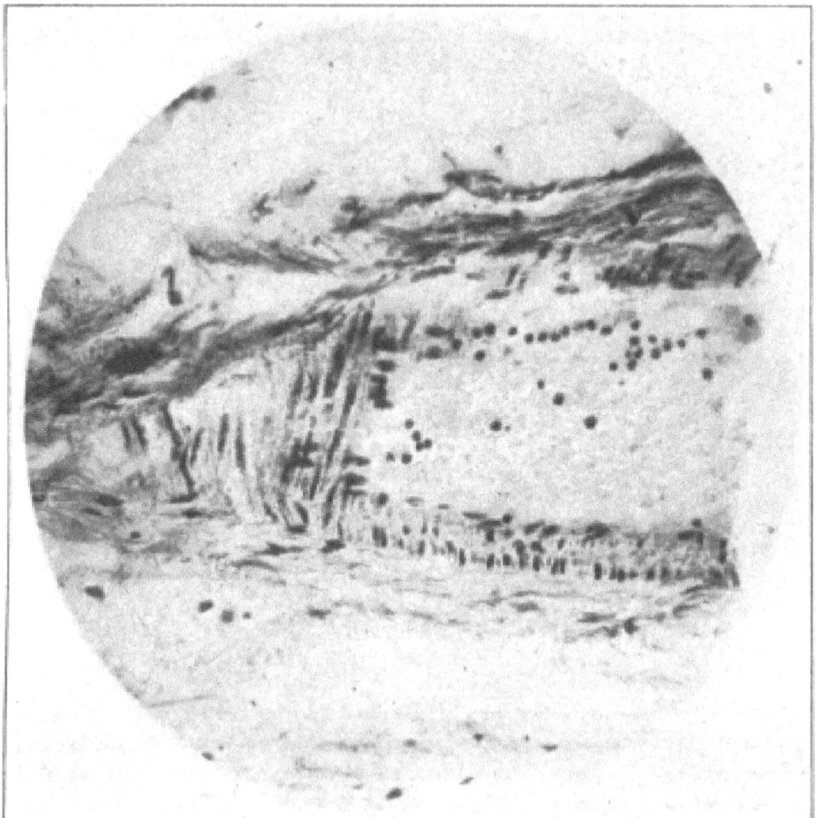

Fig. 44.—Section of the Artery from the Area of Subcutaneous Hemorrhage Shown in Fig. 42. Note the mural aggregation of leukocytes.

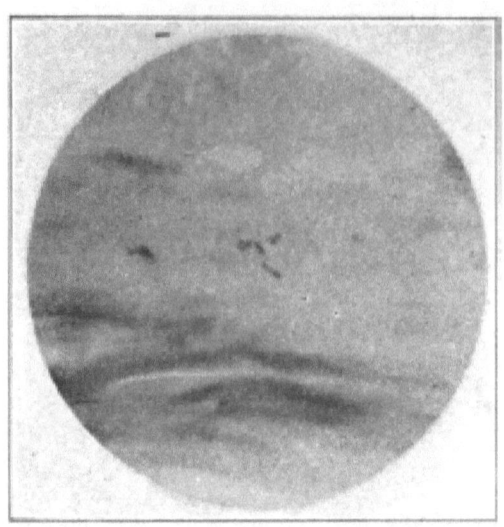

FIG. 45.—DIPLOBACILLI IN THE WALL OF ARTERY SHOWN IN FIG. 44.

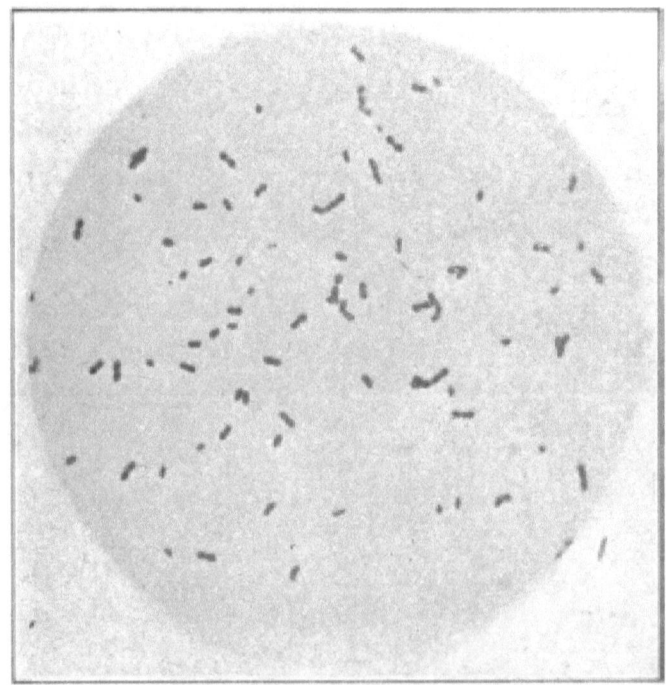

FIG. 46.—PHOTOMICROGRAPH OF 24 HOUR CULTURE IN ASCITES-DEXTROSE-BROTH OF A STREPTOCOCCUS ISOLATED FROM THE SPINAL FLUID OF A RABBIT WHICH SHOWED HERPES AFTER THE INTRAVENOUS INJECTION OF STREPTOCOCCUS CULTURE FROM THE TONSIL OF A MAN WHO SUFFERED WITH HERPES ZOSTER. The morphology is quite characteristic of the strains from herpes zoster.

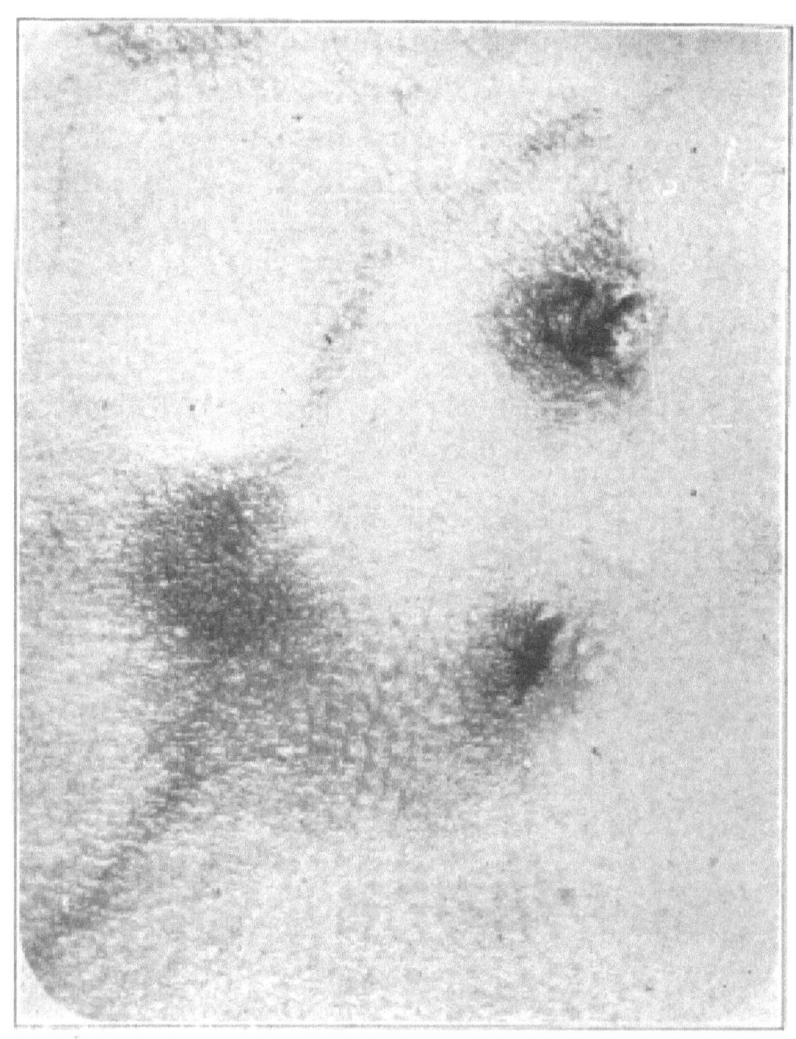

Fig. 47.—Herpes as Seen on Under Surface of the Skin Over the Lower Right Thoracic Region of a Rabbit 24 Hours After an Intravenous Injection of Streptococcus Shown in Fig. 46.

patients at the Presbyterian Hospital, suffering from erythema nodosum, has been followed with relief over periods of sufficient length of time to clinically prove the etiologic relations of the focus of infection to the systemic condition.

HERPES

It has long been known that herpetic eruptions may be induced in animals and that like lesions occur in man

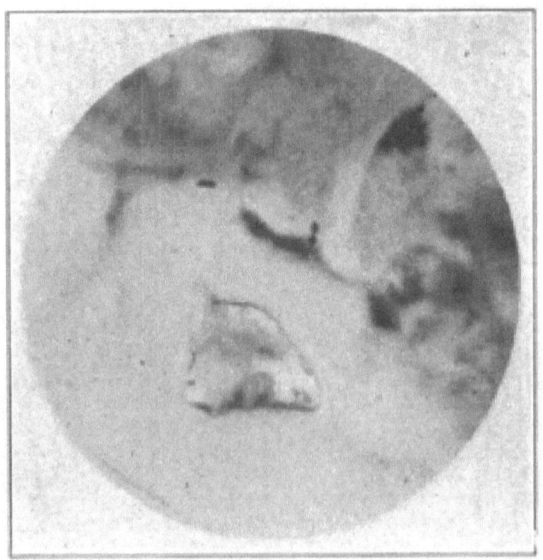

Fig. 48.—Diplococci in the Hemorrhagic Spinal Ganglion Corresponding with the Area of Herpes Shown in Fig. 47. Gram-Weigert stain.

from injury or infection of the ganglia on the sensory root of the cranial and of the spinal nerves. That herpes zoster may be the result of specific infection of the ganglia of the posterior roots of the spinal nerves and the etiologic infectious microörganisms may be isolated from the infected tonsils and other foci has been demonstrated with patients in our clinic. With these strains

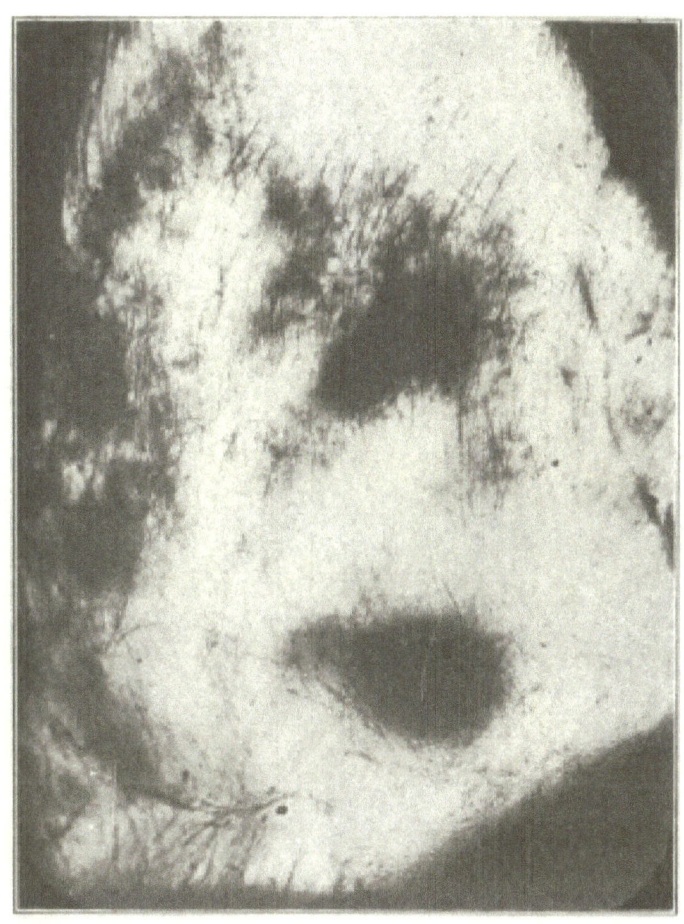

Fig. 49.—Herpes of the Skin of the Inner and Upper Aspect of Right Thigh of a Rabbit 48 Hours After Intravenous Injection of Streptococcus from the Tonsil of a Patient Suffering with Herpes Zoster.

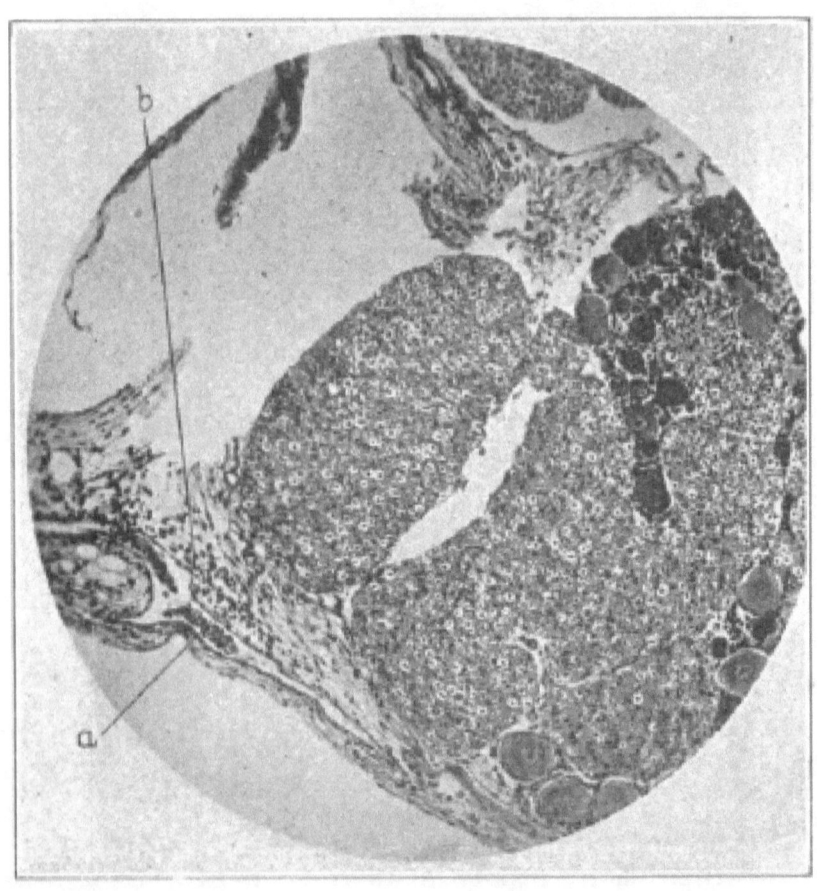

Fig. 50.—Thrombosis of a Vein (a) and Paravascular Infiltration (b) of the Posterior Spinal Root Adjacent to the Ganglion Within the Dura Corresponding to the Area of Herpes Shown in Fig. 49.

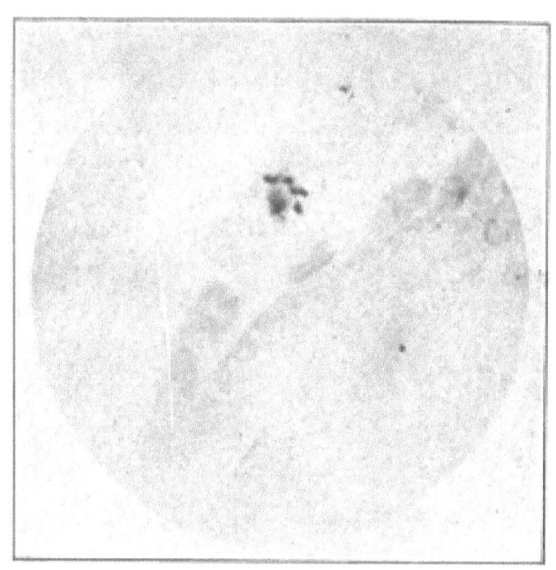

FIG. 51.—DIPLOCOCCI IN LEUKOCYTES WITHIN A THROMBOSED VEIN SHOWN IN FIG. 50. Gram-Weigert stain.

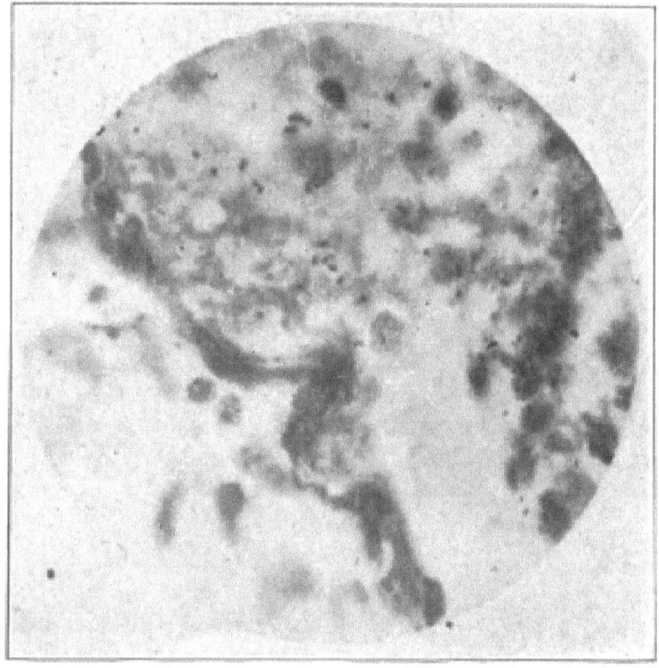

FIG. 52.—DIPLOCOCCI IN HEMORRHAGIC AND INFILTRATED AREA SHOWN IN FIG. 53. Gram-Weigert stain.

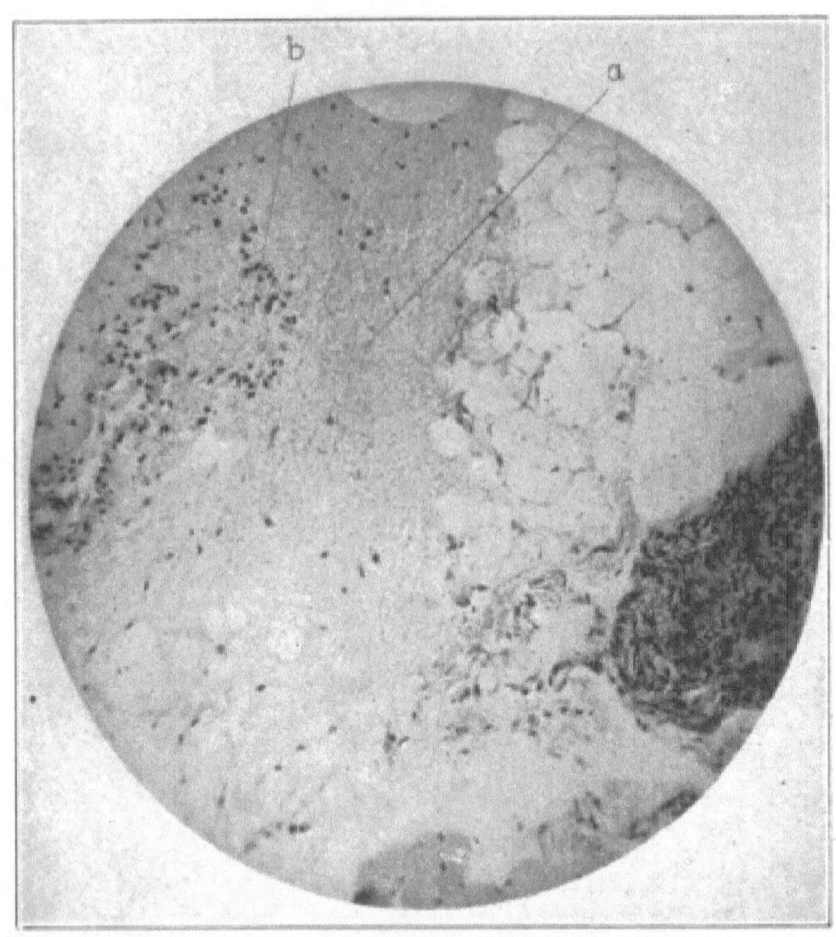

Fig. 53.—Marked Hemorrhage (a) and Leukocytic Infiltration (b)
Surrounding the Lumbar Nerve Just Outside the Spinal Canal
Corresponding to the Area of Herpes Shown in Fig. 49.

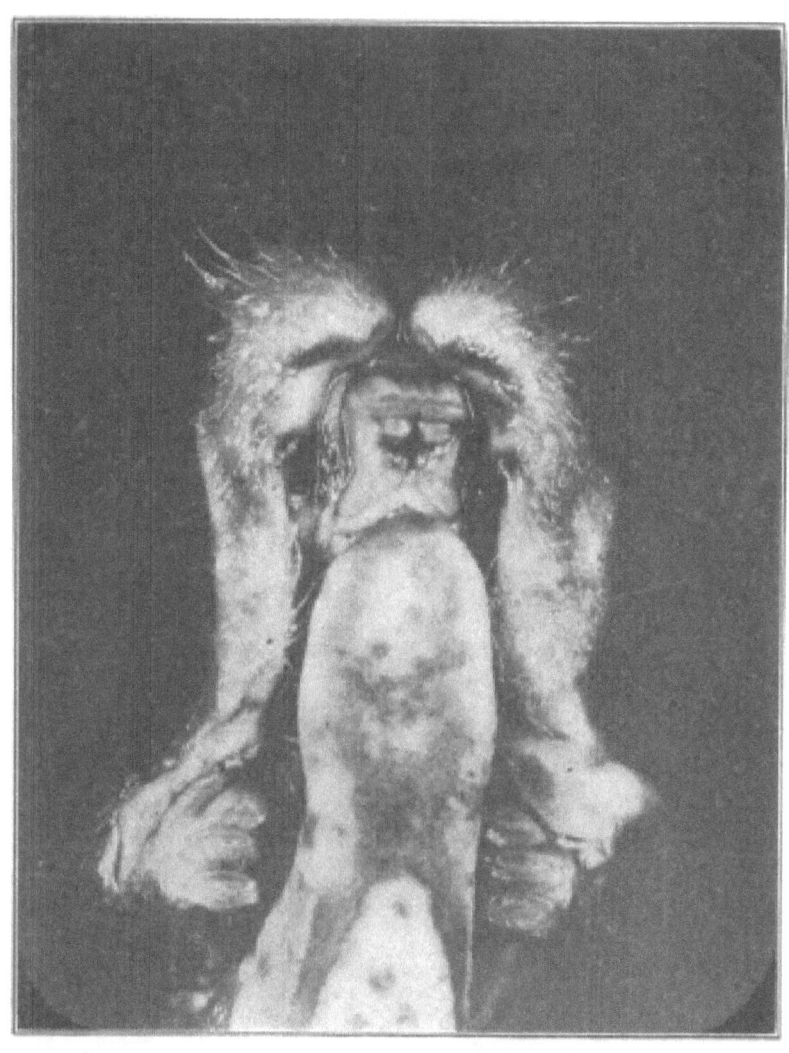

FIG. 54.—HERPES OF TONGUE, MUCOUS MEMBRANE ABOUT TEETH AND LIPS OF RABBIT 24 HOURS AFTER INTRAVENOUS INJECTION OF STREPTOCOCCUS FROM THE TONSIL IN RECURRING HERPES.

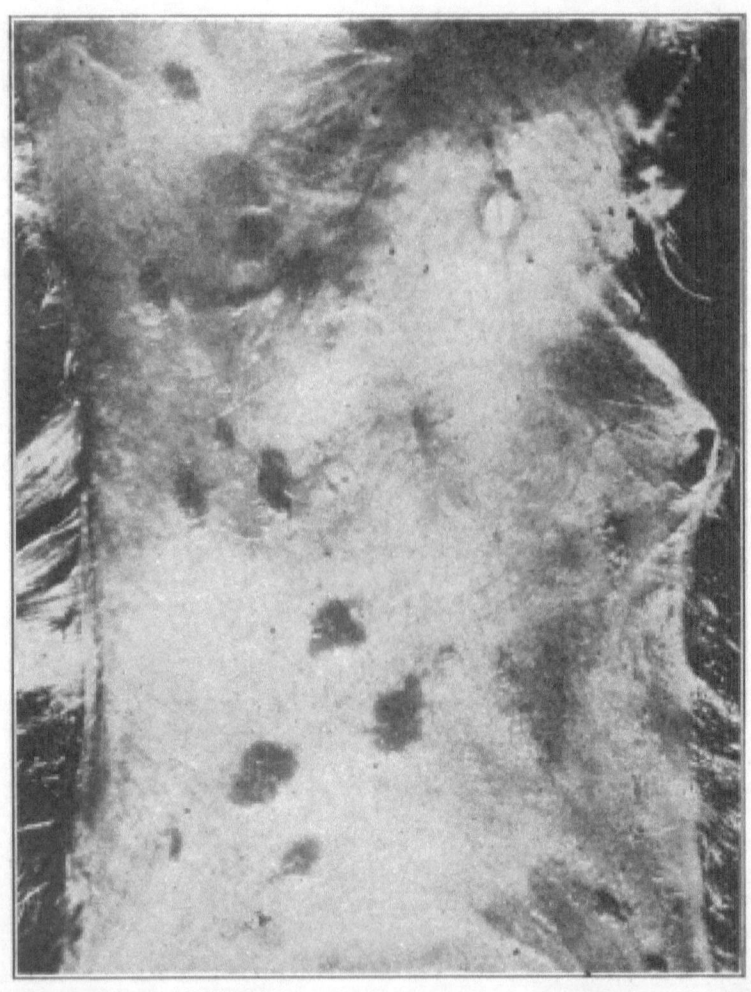

Fig. 55.—Herpes of Skin of Left Side of Face of a Rabbit 72 Hours After an Intravenous Injection of Streptococcus from the Tonsil in Herpes Zoster.

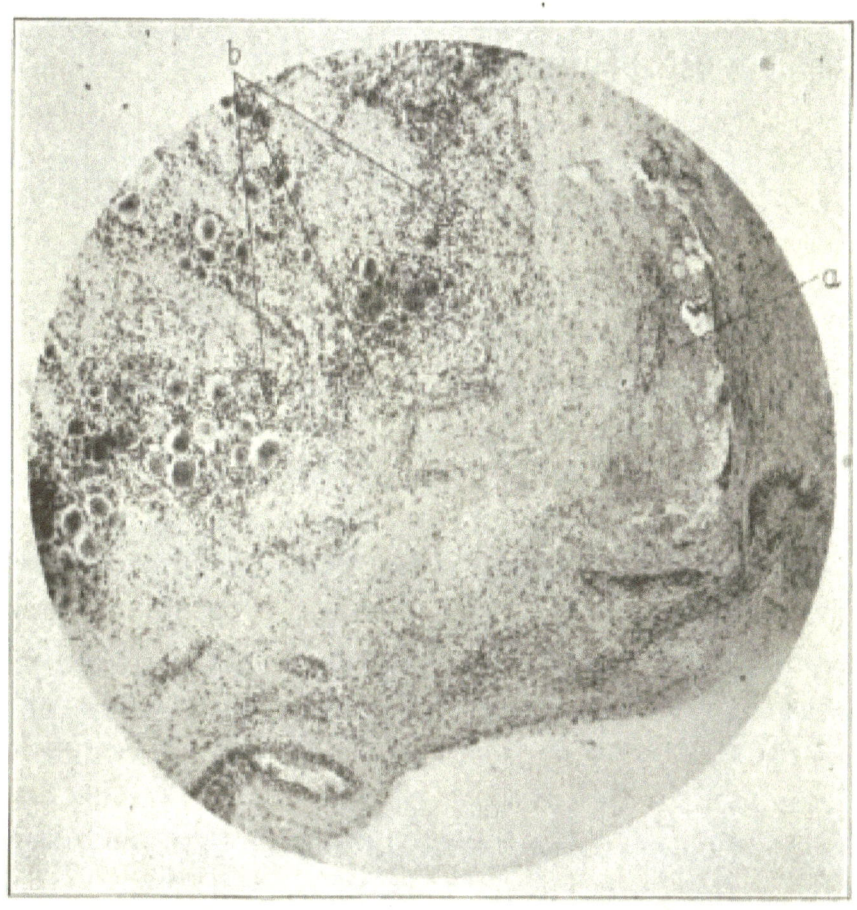

FIG. 56.—HEMORRHAGE (A) AND ROUND CELL INFILTRATION (B) OF THE GASSERIAN GANGLION OF DOG WITH MARKED HERPES OF THE LIP 48 HOURS AFTER AN INTRAVENOUS INJECTION OF STREPTOCOCCUS FROM THE TONSIL IN A PATIENT WITH LOBAR PNEUMONIA AND MARKED HERPES OF THE LIP AND CHEEK.

of the isolated bacteria, herpes zoster has been produced
in intravenously injected animals and the streptococci
have been recovered from the posterior root ganglia of
the inoculated animals.

SPINAL MYELITIS

A recent interesting clinical observation and its related laboratory experiments as made by Rosenow is
worthy of record. A young man suffered for three
years from the mild but typical symptoms of spinal insular sclerosis. When he was admitted to the hospital,
he suffered from ataxia of gait and station, greatly in-
increased knee kicks, slight nystagmus, but no intention
tremor, and his spinal fluid was negative both as
to abnormal cells and the serum tests. He had
periods of improvement and of worse conditions
associated with marked vertigo and falls without
unconsciousness. He had suffered from chronic tonsillitis for years. With a consideration of the possibility of a relation of focal infection to the condition and
as no other site of infection could be located, the tonsils
were enucleated. The streptococci isolated from the tonsillar tissue, chiefly a strain of the green forming type,
was intravenously injected into two dogs. In both
animals focal hemorrhages were produced in the spinal
cord and the development of ataxic gait and partial loss
of power in all four extremities. From the focal softened areas of the spinal cord a like strain of streptococci was recovered.

The infectious etiology of focal hemorrhage and softening of the cerebrospinal axis has been recognized for

a long time. The possibility that the condition may arise from a focus of infection is suggested by the observation and experiment just mentioned.

ACUTE OSTEOMYELITIS

Acute osteomyelitis is often ascribed to injury usually involving the extremities. There can be no question that the infectious organisms, usually tubercle bacilli, streptococci and staphylococci, gain entrance into the blood stream from foci in the head or lymph nodes and that under certain conditions of increased virulence and of lessened resistance upon the part of local tissues due to injury of the bones, single or multiple osteomyelitis may occur. Kretz (25) records clinical observation in support of the focal origin of osteomyelitis.

THYROIDITIS

Thyroiditis is probably a much more frequent event than has been heretofore noted. I have already called attention to the frequency with which thyroiditis occurs in rheumatism. Vincent (31) has shown the incidence of 50 to 80 per cent. of swelling and tenderness of the thyroid gland in the course of acute rheumatic fever. There can be no question, too, that infection of the gland occurs in other general infections. It also occurs from focal infection about the mouth, throat, and nose. We have observed many instances of thyroid enlargement, usually of chronic type, associated with evidences of thyroid intoxication in many young women patients with focal infection in the form of alveolar abscess, tonsillitis and sinusitis.

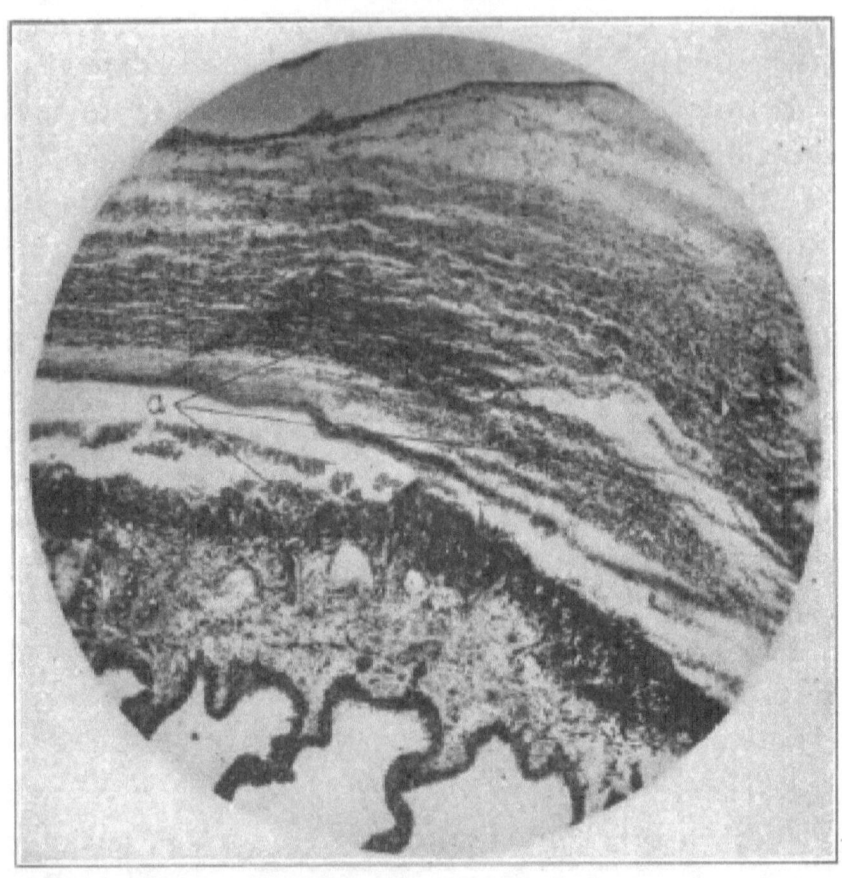

Fig. 57.—Section of Iris and Ciliary Body of Rabbit Showing Marked Leukocytic Infiltration (a) 4 Days After Intravenous Injection of Streptococci from Rheumatic Fever.

IRIDOCYCLITIS

Iritis is not an unusual event in rheumatism, syphilis and some other general infectious diseases. When acute or subacute iritis occurs alone the cause has been ascribed to infection, toxins, anaphylaxis and to faulty

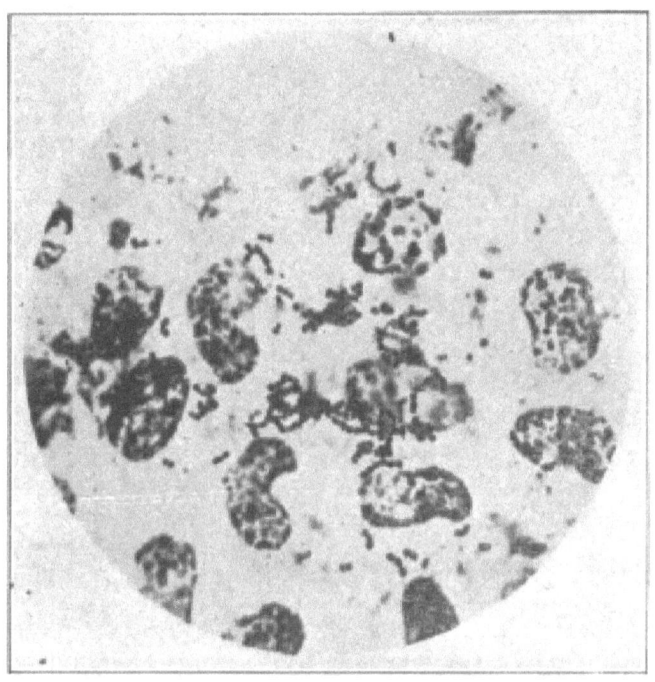

Fig. 58.—Photomicrograph of Streptococci in Area of Infiltration Shown in Fig. 57. Gram-Weigert stain.

metabolism. That infection plays a much more constant part in the causation of iritis is apparent from the experimental work of Rosenow (8), Irons and Brown and others. Strains of streptococci in foci of infection of the teeth, tonsils and sinuses have an unquestionable relation to iridocyclitis alone as well as when the eye infection is associated with rheumatic fever, chorea, syphilis and other acute general diseases.

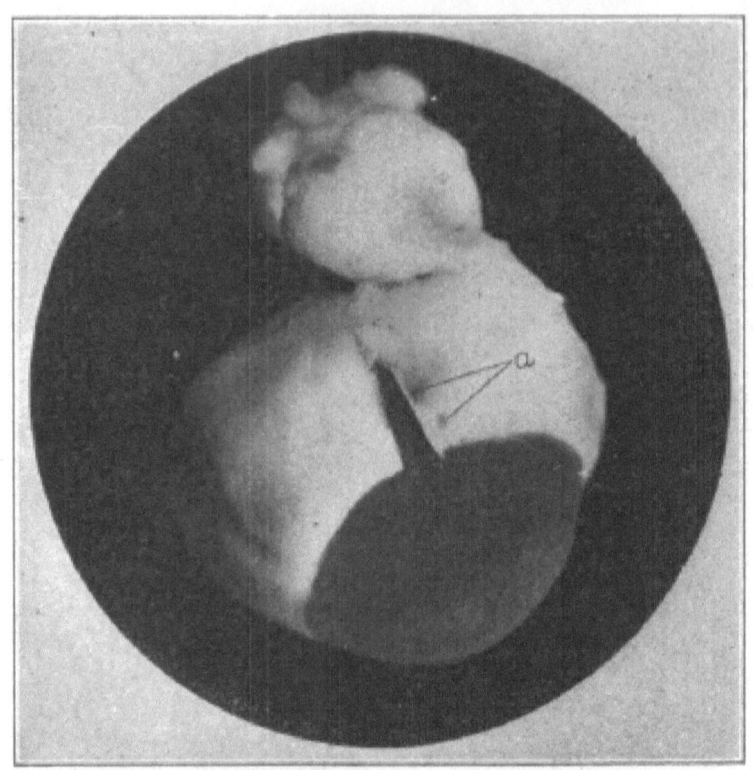

FIG. 59.—LOCALIZED HEMORRHAGES (A) IN THE SCLERA NEAR THE LIMBUS AND AT THE ATTACHMENT OF THE EXTERNAL RECTUS MUSCLE OF RABBIT 48 HOURS AFTER INTRAVENOUS INJECTION OF STREPTOCOCCI FROM PUˢ POCKET OF TONSIL.

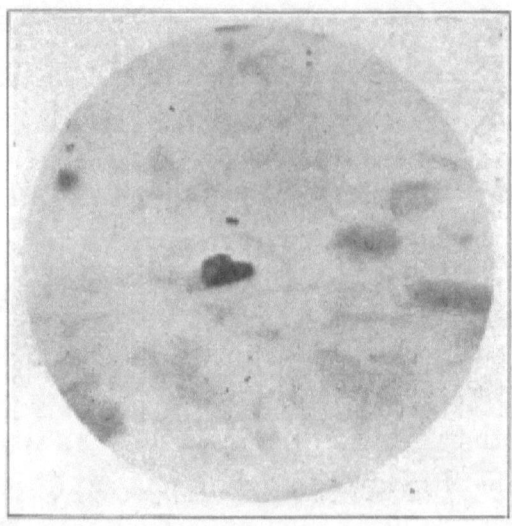

FIG. 60.—DIPLOCOCCUS ADJACENT TO AREA OF HEMORRHAGE SHOWN IN FIG. 59.

LECTURE IV

CHRONIC DISEASES RELATED TO FOCAL INFECTION

CHRONIC INFECTIOUS ARTHRITIS

Under the classification of chronic infectious arthritis our present knowledge justifies the consideration of chronic arthritis which may be due to various forms of pathogenic bacteria. Investigation has shown that a strain of the streptococcus, gonococcus, tubercle bacillus, bacillus typhosus and spirocheta pallida are the most common infectious causes of chronic arthritis. When other bacteria are found in the infected tissues of chronic arthritis and myositis, they may have etiologic relations to the condition, but are probably present in the tissues as a mixed infection or purely as parasites.

We shall confine the subject to streptococcus, gonococcus and tuberculous joint infections because of the usual focal origin. The deformities which occur in chronic arthritis due to the streptococcus and to the gonococcus do not differ essentially because the morbid anatomical changes which are produced in the chronic type of infection due to the streptococcus and to the gonococcus are essentially the same.

In both instances the mode of infection is hematogenous and from a focal infection. In both the obstruction due to endothelial proliferation or embolism in the small arteries due to the hematogenous mode of infection is practically the same. In both types of chronic infection the virulence of the invading organisms is not high. Consequently the tissue reactions excited by the organisms is much less than in the more virulent type of streptococcus and gonococcus. Consequently instead of the production of a positive chemotaxis with purulent exuda:.s at the point óf infection as with local infections due to the streptococcus pyogenes and virulent types of gonococcus, there is in these chronic conditions a tendency to fibrinoplastic exudate and an attempt to wall off an area of infection. The variation in the virulency of the organisms which produce the chronic types may result in serofibrinous exudates in joints and tendon sheaths and to small hemorrhages in subserous tissues and in muscles. The low virulency of the organism, the embolic mode of infection of the tissues, the resulting tissue reaction, all tend to lessen the blood supply of the infected tissues through the partial obliteration and destruction of small blood vessels. In consequence there is a lessened blood supply and oxygenation of the tissues which results in marked malnutrition. Malnutrition leads to secondary metabolic changes resulting in either hyperplastic or atrophic changes in all joint structures, tendons and muscles. These changes have been well described by Nichols and Richardson (41) as both proliferative or hypertrophic and degenerative or atrophic arthritis. Because of these morbid changes, deformities result from muscular contraction and from the changes which occur in the bones, cartilage and other structures entering into the joints.

Present knowledge is in accord with Nichols and Richardson in the statement they make that morbid changes both proliferative and degenerative of joint tissue cannot be differentiated etiologically.

If one considers that the infection of joint tissue is hematogenous and that a sufficient dose of infectious organisms in the blood stream may reach the peri-articular tissue or deeper tissue of the joint—that is, the end arteries in the subcapsular tissues—or through the nutrient arteries and involve the medulla of the epiphysis, one can harmonize the morbid anatomical changes which have been so clearly described by Nichols and Richardson.

The reaction set up in the tissues of the external joint structures in the subcapsular region and in the medulla of the bone will depend in all probability upon the virulence of the infectious microörganisms and upon the resistance of the general body structures and of the joint tissues. They may be either proliferative with virulent bacteria, especially in young or normal individuals, and necessarily the reaction will be less, or more degenerative in kind in the joint tissues of individuals, which are poor because of age, trauma and other conditions which lessen the vitality of tissue.

Continued doses of infection from the focus would necessarily add to the changes described in the joint tissue. The repeated hematogenous infection destroys more blood vessels, again and again traumatizes the infected tissue and continuously lessens the oxygen supply.

We now know that in chronic arthritis infectious

organisms, whether streptococci or gonococci, have a relatively low virulence. Of course the degree of virulence varies and consequently the proliferative and degenerative changes especially vary in different individuals.

With continued infection of the tissues malnutrition necessarily increases, for the reasons named, and this necessarily leads to retrograde metabolism.

Whether the retrograde metabolism is due solely to the malnutritions or whether it is also due in part to irritants in the tissues of bacterial or biochemic origin, does not in any way alter the principles outlined. Therefore, the proper understanding of chronic infectious arthritis involves an understanding of the following principles:

(1) The infection of the joints, muscles and other involved tissues with pathogenic organisms which usually are members of the streptococcus group and the gonococcus which are of relatively low virulence; (2) a hematogenous infection with embolism with resulting injury of blood vessels and small hemorrhages into the infected tissues; (3) lessened blood supply and oxygenation and consequent relative starvation of the infected tissues and dependent upon the malnutrition, favorable conditions for the continued life and multiplication of the infectious organisms, and finally (4) retrograde metabolism due to the malnutrition.

In the chronic infections due to the streptococcus, chronic arthritis may occur alone or associated with chronic myositis and chronic myositis may also occur alone involving single or groups of muscles. In chronic gonococcus arthritis the muscles are rarely, if ever, involved. Tenovaginitis is, however, more apt to occur than in chronic streptococcus infection.

Various anatomical types of chronic infectious arthritis may occur, which doubtless depends upon the degree of bacteriemia, the degree of virulence of the infectious organisms, the resistance of the tissues and the fact that the mode of infection is hematogenous. Consequently we may have a peri-arthritis, a synovitis, an osteo-arthritis or a panarthritis. Any or all of these types may exist in the same individual. The primary infection may be severe enough to simulate acute rheumatic fever or mild rheumatic fever. Usually the disease begins insidiously, but there may be in many patients periods of increase in temperature usually of a febrile type. There is always a great deal of soreness of the infected tissues which is aggravated by anything which disturbs the general or local circulation, as chilling the body, fatigue and general nervous irritability. Because of the varying degrees of activity of the focus there may be reinfection from time to time of the tissues, joints, muscles, etc., with consequent aggravation of the symptoms. Usually there is but little pain excepting with exercise of the involved organs. Chronic gonorrheal arthritis is more apt to involve the intervertebral joints and ligaments, the sacroiliac, sternoclavicular and temporomaxillary joints than the streptococcus, but inasmuch as the streptococcus may also infect the four named joints, involvement of them does not necessarily indicate a gonococcus infection. Chronic infectious myositis which may occur as a part of the chronic streptococcus arthritis or alone, is associated with shortening of the muscle bundles due to the embolic infection with subsequent hemorrhage and connective tissue proliferation. At the time of infection there is usually tenderness and pain when an attempt is made to contract the muscles. When at rest there is usually no discomfort. There is apparently an elective affinity of the infectious organism for certain muscles, notably the masseters, the biceps humeri, the hamstrings, the anterior tibial and erector spinae groups. Other muscles are sometimes involved and in some instances practically all skeletal muscles are included in the infection.

In all of these chronic types of arthritis and myositis there may be general debility with anemia, emaciation and nervous irritability due to the long continued infection. Often these general conditions are aggravated by methods of treatment, in starvation diets and purges which weaken the patient and by the overuse of drugs. In recent years the irrational use of vaccines and of toxic extracts of bacteria has added to the miserable condition of the patients.

These general weakening influences add to the conditions which promote retrograde metabolism in the infected tissues, so that in the patients who present the worst type of the condition there is a tendency to such a degree of retrograde metabolism that the connective tissue group comprising aponeurosis, tendons and cartilage is changed into bone.

Chronic tuberculous arthritis is always associated with focal or with general tuberculosis. It practically always occurs as an osteomyelitis usually involving the epiphysis. The evolution of the tuberculous process in the epiphysis leads to infection of the joint with its characteristic morbid anatomy. Tuberculous tenovaginitis is usually a secondary infection from the periarticular tissues, but may occur alone.

Spondylitis due to the typhoid bacillus probably causes the same anatomical type as the gonococcus and streptococcus.

Infectious neuritis or perineuritis due to a focus of infection may occur alone or as a part of chronic arthritis and myositis or with myositis without arthritis. Usually the condition is a perineuritis. The nerves most often involved are branches of the brachial plexus and the sciatic trunks. Focal infection about the teeth, tonsils and sinuses is a frequent cause of neuritis. The gonococcus may be the cause of neuritis or perineuritis.

CHRONIC INFECTIOUS NEPHRITIS

Chronic infectious nephritis due to focal infection is very common. Probably it has first existed as a subacute infectious nephritis and not infrequently occurs as a hematogenous infection of the kidney from some focus resulting in anatomical changes of various degrees. Chronic infectious nephritis, like the subacute and acute types, is usually due to strains of the streptococcus which have a specific elective affinity for the kidney. This specific affinity may be attained in the focus of infection. If the bacteriemia due to focal infection is severe, undoubtedly nephritis either acute or chronic may result from bacteria which have only general pathologic virulence. LeCount and Jackson (35) state that

the most important result of their work was the experimental production of alterations, essentially subacute
and quite like the acute interstitial nephritis in human
kidneys, caused by the acute infectious diseases, com-

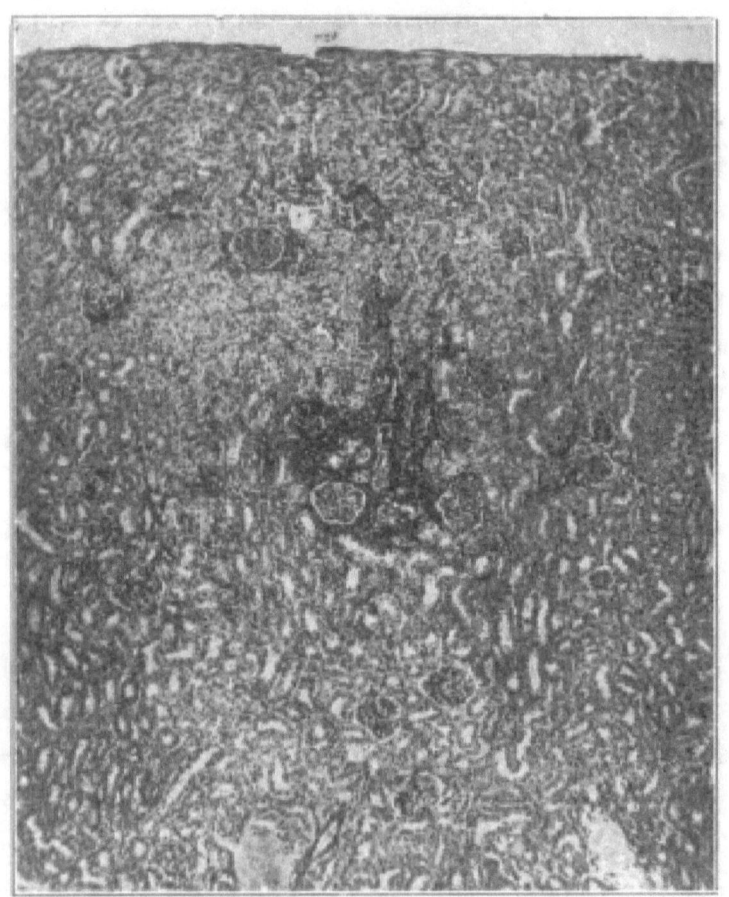

FIG. 61.—A TYPICAL SUBACUTE FOCAL LESION IN THE CORTEX. X 200 (after
LeCount and Jackson, Jour. Inf. Dis.).

plicated by or due to streptococcus infection. Of the
rabbits inoculated, eight, or 25 per cent. of the thirty-
three which died or were killed within the first two
weeks, showed chronic changes in the kidneys, while fifteen, or 62. 5 per cent., of twenty-four rabbits which lived

from fifteen to one hundred and eighty-six days, showed chronic kidney changes. They conclude, therefore, that chronic lesions of the kidney of a part of the inoculated

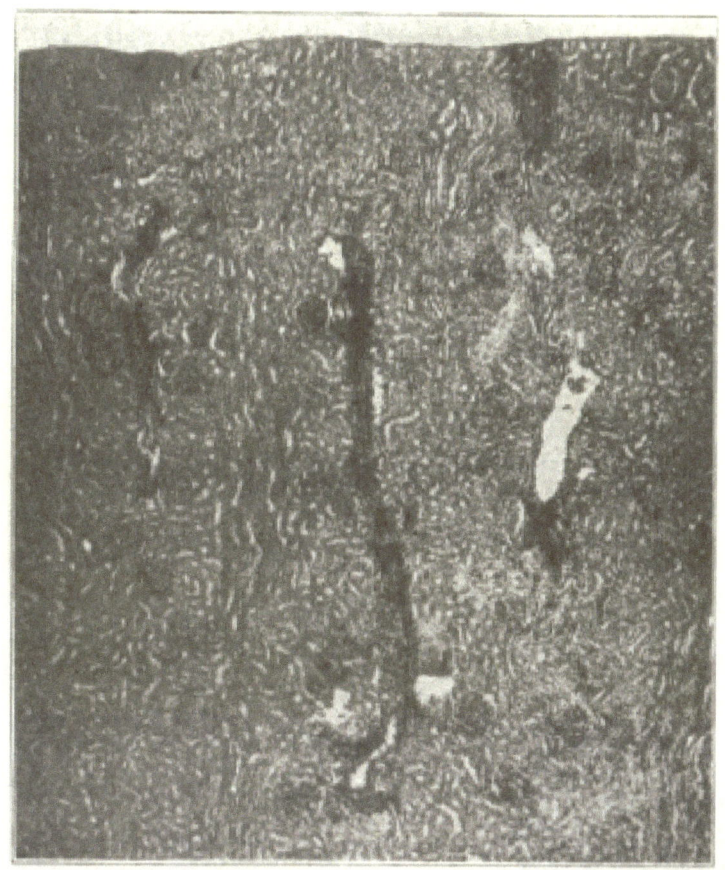

Fig. 62.—An Interlobular Vein Surrounded by Lymphocytes and Plasma Cells. From the kidney of rabbit dying 42 days after inoculation. X 35 (after LeCount and Jackson, Jour. Inf. Dis.).

rabbits resulted from the subacute nephritis caused by the streptococci intravenously injected.

Ophüls (55) concludes that chronic nephritis is usually of infectious origin. Klotz (54) states that a form of acute interstitial nephritis induced in animals by the inoculation with strains of streptococci subsequently gives rise to a renal sclerosis of the type known as chronic interstitial nephritis. He believes that a similar process is common in man.

In an article on the relation of focal infection to nephritis, we gave the clinical history of a young woman who suffered with hemorrhagic nephritis apparently due to badly infected tonsils. After enucleation of the tonsils there was great improvement of the renal condition and a restoration to apparent health. Occasionally, slight albuminuria with the presence of hyalogranular casts occurred. After one year evidences of chronic interstitial nephritis became constant and three years following the removal of the tonsils and the greatly improved condition, the patient died of renal intoxication associated with a high degree of hypertension.

Every clinician of experience has observed patients over long periods of time who have presented primarily evidences of acute or subacute nephritis of infectious origin and who have finally succumbed to chronic nephritis. That a focal infection may be the source of the kidney lesions and may lead to a chronic irreparable renal disease must be emphasized. Early removal of the etiologic focus may prevent further anatomical insult of the kidneys and preserve renal function and life.

CHRONIC CHOLECYSTITIS

Chronic cholecystitis with or without gall-stones is the result of acute infection as a rule. As we have seen, this may be due to hematogenous streptococcus infec-

tion. The streptococci, which lodge in the small area
of the fundus of the gall-bladder at the terminus of a
blood vessel. may cause hemorrhage and exciting tissue

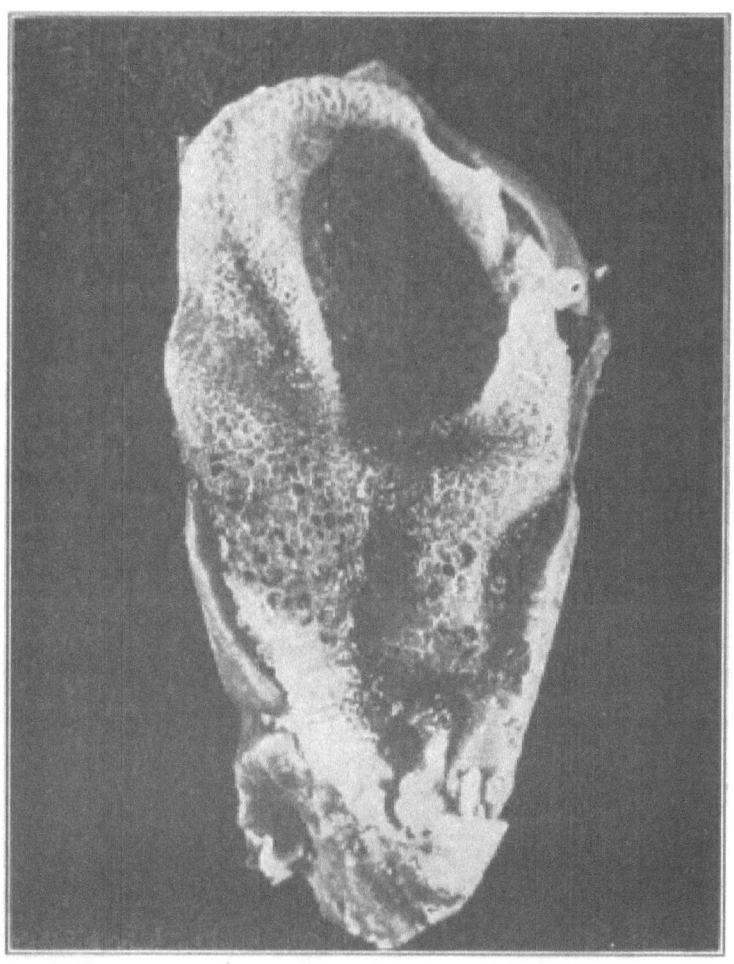

Fig. 63.—Cholectstitis and Cholelithiasis in Dog Ten Days After Intravenous Injection of Streptococcus from Center of Gall-Stone from Human Gall-Bladder. Note the black stones imbedded in the edematous mucous membrane.

reaction which weakens the gall-bladder wall and may
rupture into the cyst. If the infectious organism is of
high virulency, acute purulent cholecystitis may occur

or with a less virulent type the infection will be much
less in degree. If unoperated at the time of the acute
or subacute attack, gall-stones may form in the chronically infected gall-bladder. As long as the focal site
exists reinfection may lead to subsequent acute or subacute attacks of cholecystitis.

As shown by Rosenow (8) the strain of streptococcus, which seems to acquire an affinity for the tissue
of the gall-bladder, has a coincident affinity for muscles
particularly of the myocardium, and in confirmation
clinicians have noted evidences of myocardial weakness
in patients who suffer from chronic cholecystitis.

CHRONIC PEPTIC ULCER

Chronic peptic ulcers of the stomach and duodenum
are doubtless the sequence of acute ulceration and we
have already noted the mode of infection in acute ulcer

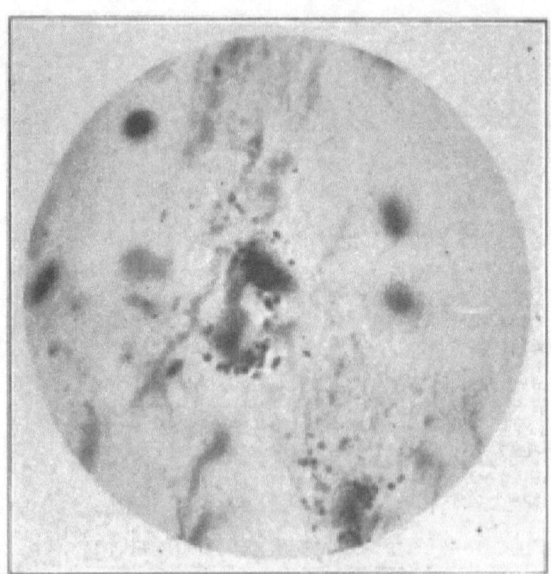

FIG. 64.—STREPTOCOCCI AND LEUKOCYTIC INFILTRATION IN PERITONEAL COAT
IN PERFORATING ULCER OF THE STOMACH OF MAN.

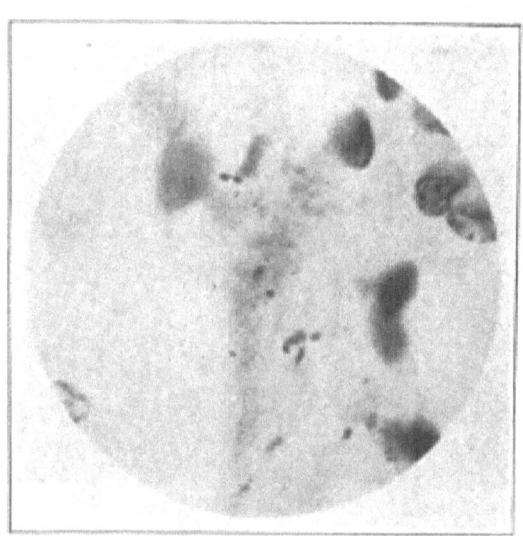

FIG. 65.—STREPTOCOCCI IN PERITONEAL COAT OF ULCER OF STOMACH IN
RABBIT 5 DAYS AFTER INTRAVENOUS INJECTION OF STREPTOCOCCI FROM
PERFORATING ULCER OF STOMACH IN MAN SHOWN IN FIG. 64.

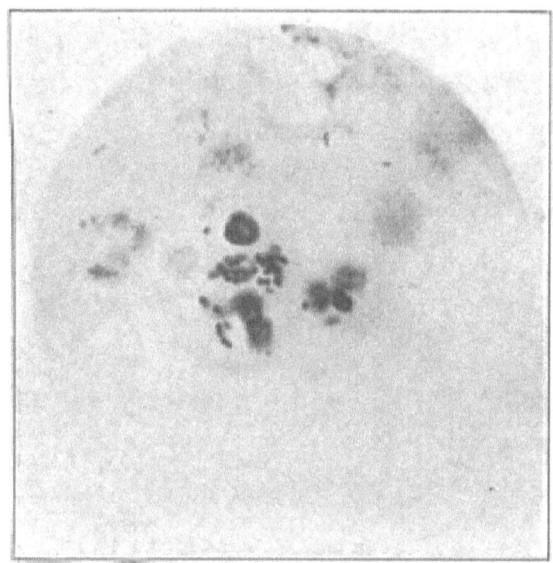

FIG. 66.—STREPTOCOCCI AND LEUKOCYTIC INFILTRATION IN CHRONIC ULCER
OF MAN WITH ACUTE EXACERBATION SHORTLY BEFORE OPERATION.

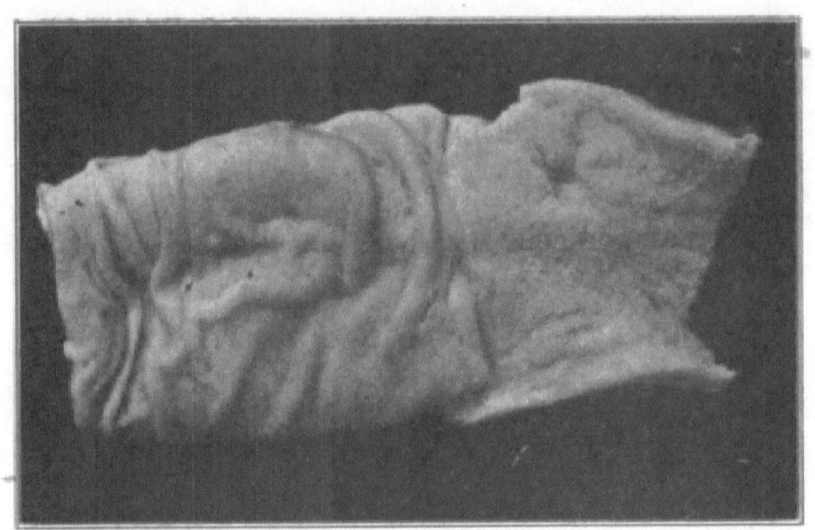

FIG. 67. CHRONIC ULCER OF DUODENUM OF DOG 13 WEEKS AFTER SINGLE
INTRAVENOUS INJECTION OF STREPTOCOCCUS FROM ULCER OF THE DUO-
DENUM OF MAN.

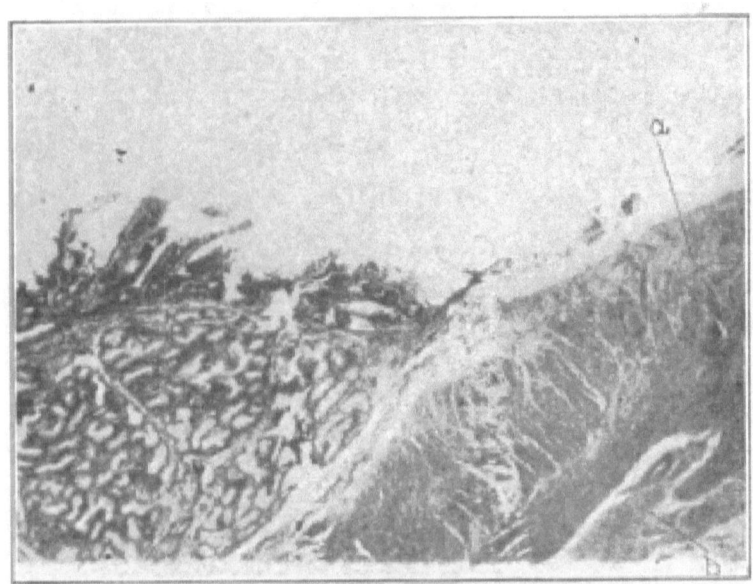

FIG. 68.—CHRONIC ULCER OF DUODENUM OF DOG 13 WEEKS AFTER A SINGLE
INTRAVENOUS INJECTION OF STREPTOCOCCUS FROM HUMAN ULCER. Note
the displacement of muscular layer (a) by connective tissue and the
thickened peritoneal coat (b).

and the immediate morbid tissue changes which occur. In the hematogenous embolic infection of the stomach with a strain of the streptococcus which has an elective affinity for the stomach wall, a local submucous hemorrhage occurs.   In consequence of the hemorrhage and infection, anemic necrosis results with consequent lessened resistance and the necrosed tissues of this small area are digested by the gastric juice.   The continued infection of the tissues around the acute ulcer prevents the healing of the mucous membrane of the stomach in all probability, for it is well known that uninfected wounds of the stomach readily heal.   The continued action of the gastric juice upon the ulcer base results in the characteristic anatomical picture of chronic peptic ulcer.

CHRONIC INFECTIOUS ENDOCARDITIS

In 1903 Schottmüller (10) reported the isolation of a green-forming streptococcus in blood agar plates from the blood of patients suffering from endocarditis. This report was made in connection with the investigation which Schottmüller was at that time making of the growth characteristics of streptococci upon blood agar. He called this green-producing microörganism streptococcus viridans.   Its low virluency led also to the name, streptococcus mitior.

The character of the endocarditis in which the streptococcus viridans seemed to be the infectious agent has proved to be one of a paradoxical nature in the sense that the clinical course, in the early stages, is frequently very mild and the patient is able often to be up and about, even attending to ordinary affairs of life, but it is progressive and in a few weeks or months, sometimes as late as a year and a half, the patient usually succumbs to the disease.

It is, therefore, a malignant type of endocarditis although usually chronic in its clinical course. As I have before stated the streptococcus viridans endocarditis may sometimes be very acute and associated with a septic type of temperature with a very high maximum and low minimum temperature, and may run its entire clinical course within two or three weeks. During the last few years since routine blood cultures have been made, the frequent incidence of this disease has become noted. Osler (17), Horder (18), Libman (20), Lenhartz (22) and others have reported a series of patients suffering from what they have termed chronic infectious endocarditis, infective endocarditis, subacute infective endocarditis, subacute bacterial endocarditis and the report which Rosenow and Billings made was under the title of "chronic pneumococcus endocarditis."

The characteristics of this type of malignant endocarditis are usually a mild clinical course in which the patient may complain of lessened strength and endurance; usually a poor appetite; more or less dyspnoea of exertion; slight to severe chills and fever in periods often mistaken for malaria; cough, in some cases with more or less expectoration, often with a septic type of fever mistaken for tuberculosis, and in severe grades sometimes treated for mild typhoid fever. The majority of these patients have suffered at some time from rheumatism and endocarditis or from endocarditis alone and upon examination it is usual to find the evidences of old valvular disease with varying conditions as to the heart muscle. Those patients who have not previously suffered from endocarditis may present no heart murmurs or other evidence of heart involvement. While in bed the temperature is usually a mildly febrile one of septic type and there may be rigors amounting at times to severe chills. Sooner or later with involvement of the left heart there are evidences of embolism in petechia of the skin and elsewhere. Frequently there are infarcts of the spleen manifested by enlargement and tenderness of that organ. Infarcts of the kidney manifested by hematuria usually microscopic (See Baehr (23) and Lohlein (24)), embolism of brain with varying degrees of sensory or motor disturbance and in some patients embolism of sufficient size of the arteries of the extremities to obliterate the pulse below the site of the embolus and to cause gangrene of the extremities. Mycotic aneurism may occur usually situated in the smaller arteries. Death supervenes with severe embolism of the brain or from exhaustion with mixed infection. The duration may be from two to three weeks in the really acute types of the disease and may last for eighteen or more months.

The streptococcus viridans may be isolated from the blood and is characterized by the fact that in culture media it soon loses its affinity for the heart and may be converted, as shown in the immunological studies of Rosenow (8), into any of the other types of the members of the streptococcus-pneumococcus group.

The lesion of the heart in streptococcus viridans endocarditis is characterized by the growth of massive vegetations upon the valves and upon the mural endocardium. (See Figs. 9 and 10.) It is not usually attended with ulcerations, but there is an enormous deposit of thrombus in the vegetations which serves as a rich culture medium for the invading organism and also because of the size and friability of the vegetations and the thrombus formation is a ready source for the dissemination of emboli of all sizes through the systemic vessels.

It is a non-pus-forming organism and consequently suppuration does not follow in the tissues involved in the embolism. In rare instances the mycotic aneurism may break into the surrounding tissues and in two patients under my observation abscesses formed and a pneumococcus was obtained in pure culture therefrom, while in the blood stream was found the streptococcus viridans in pure culture.

The streptococcus viridans endocarditis is usually fatal. Streptococcus viridans bacteriemia unassociated with endocarditis, although there may be an endocardial murmur present, is not necessarily fatal. The reports of recoveries of streptococcus viridans endocarditis may be of those patients who have streptococcus viridans bacteriemia without a real endocarditis. Libman has reported recoveries, and in a series reported by Horder the mortality was not absolute. In my own experience only three patients out of more than one hundred who have had a streptococcus viridans bacteriemia have recovered from that condition. In one of these there was no recognizable heart murmur and the condition was associated with streptococcus viridans infarct of the right lung with suppuration, evacuation of abscess and recov·ery. In another, a boy of sixteen, with a systolic mitral murmur and moderate septic fever, the bacteria finally disappeared from the blood and recovery ensued with moderate mitral insufficiency fully compensated. In a third patient, a Jewess, with mitral stenosis and mod-erate septic fever of long duration mistaken before en-tering the Presbyterian Hospital for tuberculosis of the lung, the bacteriemia disappeared and five years later the patient was entirely well except for the mitral sten-osis, fully compensated.

Even with evidences of endocarditis in the last two patients described, it was not proved that there was an endocarditis of recent origin.

The character of the changes in the myocardium and valves is so serious in this disease, very much like that of the acute malignant endocarditis due to the pneumo-coccus, that one can appreciate the fatal nature of the condition.

That healing may occur though rarely cannot be doubted when one examines the heart in an accidental death with coroner's inquest where the enormous vegeta-tions can still be recognized but so infiltrated with cal-cium salts that a practical cure has resulted. This condi-tion has been noted as I have stated previously in the ob-servation of LeCount.

The focus of infection which undoubtedly causes the streptococcus viridans bacteriemia and chronic malig-nant endocarditis is often alveolar abscess. Of this we have had numerous clinical examples. Coincident cul-

tures from the alveolar abscess and from the blood
have yielded strains of streptococcus viridans. When
these nascent cultures were intravenously injected into
animals, typical endocardial lesions resulted. Doubtless a focus containing this streptococcus may be located in the tonsil or nasal sinus or elsewhere which
may be the source of the cardiac infection.

LECTURE V

FOCAL INFECTION

Prevention of focal infection is an important principle in the consideration of the treatment of the etiologic factor and the related systemic infections.

We may not hope so to modify the actions of individuals or of society that communicable diseases will disappear or that susceptibility to infection will be overcome in the evolution of a mentally and physically better developed race, for we cannot wholly prevent or abolish the marriage or procreation of the unfit; vice; alcoholic and drug addictions; poverty, unhealthful domiciliary and occupational environment; the use of contaminated food and drink; community uncleanliness, and other causes of mental and physical debility which directly diminish the natural body defenses.

The control of these debility-producing factors is a function of national, state and municipal public health bodies. Politics, greed for wealth and ignorance are influences which prevent the administration of well-established laws which, if properly enforced, would do much to abolish unhealthful conditions and disease.

As far as possible, as individuals and collectively, physicians should exert an influence to promote cleanliness of mind and body and thus lessen the incidence of focal and systemic infection. The encouragement of personal cleanliness and especially the care of the skin and its appendages, and of the mouth and throat should be a duty of the family physician. The necessity of cleansing the mouth, teeth and throat of all particles of food after eating should be taught as a prevention of local infection, decay of teeth and of general disease. When other measures fail the removal of the persistent overgrowth of lymphoid tissue, a good culture medium for bacteria, of the nasopharynx and throat should be advised. Chronically enlarged pharyngeal tonsils, which obstruct the upper respiratory tract and prevent proper ventilation and drainage, invite local infection of the mucous tracts of the head and should be totally removed.

The foregoing statements are applicable chiefly in childhood, for children are especially susceptible to infection of the tissues of the mouth, throat, nose, accessory sinuses, middle ear and mastoid cells. We know that freedom from streptococcus infection of the mucous membrane and lymphoid tissues of the head would very much lessen the incidence of rheumatism, chorea and endocarditis in children and also in adults. We may not as confidently expect to prevent acute appendicitis, peptic ulcer, cholecystitis and nephritis by these measures; still, the evidence of the etiologic relations of these dangerous local infections to focal nose, mouth and throat infection is so strong that the correction of these confined infections is rationally indicated. I do not wish to seem to be an advocate of unnecessary operations, for many operations of all kinds are irrationally performed, including the removal of overgrowth of the tonsils and other lymphoid and mucous tissues of the nose and throat. These conditions of the nose and throat may disappear with a proper hygienic management. I believe that tonsillectomy is often needlessly performed for the relief of a systemic infection, when the real focal cause is situated elsewhere. Doubtless the normal faucial tonsillar tissue has a beneficent function and uninfected, should not be molested. But too often the tonsillar tissue in children and also in some adults is a culture medium of pathogenic bacteria and as such is a constant source of danger as a portal of entry of infectious bacteria through the lymph and blood streams to the tissues of the body. Infected tonsils cannot be successfully sterilized by any known method of treatment and entire removal is the only safe procedure. If necessary a properly directed surgical treatment of the easily recognized morbid anatomical condition of the nasopharynx and nares will establish normal ventilation and drainage and lessen the incidence of middle ear, mastoid and accessory sinus disease with the resulting possible systemic involvement from these sites of focal infection. Until recently the importance of pyorrhea dentalis and alveolar abscess as an etiologic factor in systemic infection has not been recognized. Clinical and laboratory observation and research have definitely settled the question. As has been stated in the first lecture, the members of the streptococcus group, but occasionally other bacteria, are the pathogenic agents of pyorrhea which cause systemic infection. The endameba buccalis may have an etiologic relation to the pyorrhea of the teeth and alveoli, may intensify the destructive local disease and may be the agents of communicating the disease to others by direct personal contact or through fomites. The existence of focal infection of the jaws in the form of chronic alveolar abscess, without the manifestation of much discomfort, is remarkable. The condition is often not discoverable by inspection and escapes the attention of the physician and the dentist. It is only when destructive lesions of the gum, tooth and alveolus make the condition visible that a diagnosis is usually made. Properly made Röntgen ray films of the jaws will enable one to recognize the real morbid and anatomical condition. The definite recognition of the condition and the character of the mechanical dentistry which should be practiced demands the use of Röntgen ray films of the jaws. The use of emetin in the destruction of the endameba may rid the mouth temporarily of an etiologic factor of pyorrhea, but the drug does not remove the infectious bacteria in the focus, nor does it restore the periosteum of the root of the tooth without which the tooth ceases to be living bone and as a foreign body invites added and continued bacterial infection.

In a consideration of amebic dysentery, Phillips (51) states that emetin will kill the parasite in the active stage, while the drug has but little or no effect on the cysts. He suggests the hypodermic use of emetin in ten-day periods, with gradually increasing intervals, until repeated examinations finally fail to find endamebas in the stool. Inasmuch as emetin destroys endameba buccalis, the same method of management may more certainly rid the mouth of the parasite.

Dentists everywhere are interested in the better management and correction of alveolar infection. We must look to them for a treatment which will destroy the focal infection of the jaws and safeguard the individual from systemic infection. Deplorable as the loss of teeth may be, that misfortune is justified if it is necessary to obliterate the infectious focus which is a continued menace to the general health.

Malnutrition and general debility due to chronic disease, old age, and other causes may lead to focal infection of the jaws. Such foci of infection tend to add infection to already infected systemic tissues. These infectious foci, which in a way are secondary to the systemic disease causing the general debility, are just as dangerous as primary foci and should be removed.

Persistent lymph node infections which do not disappear with hygienic measures instituted to improve the defenses of the body should be surgically removed as a matter of protection against the further dissemination of tuberculosis or of some other disease from the specifically infected nodes.

The conditions which may promote infection of the gastro-intestinal tract are usually not brought to the attention of the physician until too late to use measures of prevention. Myriads of infectious bacteria are swallowed in infected food, especially milk, and in the muco pus of the nose, throat and bronchi. The gastric juice and other digestive fluids probably destroy most of these bacteria in robust individuals. The surviving microörganisms may reach the tissues of the bowel and the adjacent lymph nodes, under favorable conditions may continue to have or may attain pathogenic virulence, and cause local or systemic disease. Habitual constipation, with or without congenital or acquired anatomical deformities of the intestinal tract, may lower the natural resistance of the tissues to invasion by the bacteria of the intestine. Again the morbid anatomical conditions which favor intestinal stasis may promote increased general virulence or elective tissue affinity of the invading bacteria. Rosenow (8) has demonstrated an acquired virulence and also an elective tissue affinity for the appendix of a strain of colon bacilli isolated in cultures from the exudate and tissues in patients with appendicitis. When injected intravenously appendicitis developed in the inoculated animals. After a time the general virulence and specific tissue affinity was lost in subcultures of this strain. Beaussenat quoted by Adrian (28) was unable to produce appendicitis by the intravenous injection of ordinary strains of colon bacilli without first injuring the mucous membrane of the organ.

Infection of the digestive tract may be prevented or at any rate its incidence may be diminished very much by obliterating the sources of the mucopus in the throat and nose, which at the same time removes the foci of infection of the head, and also by avoiding infected food.

Stasis of the bowels, whether due to habitual constipation or to congenital or acquired anatomical conditions, should have a proper medical management or, if necessary, surgical treatment. I very much doubt if the removal of the entire colon is justifiable for intestinal stasis alone; certainly not to the degree practiced by some surgeons. Chronic appendicitis with lessened tissue resistance invites acute attacks, disturbs the gastric digestion and may be a focus of systemic infection. The same is true of chronic cholecystitis and especially as the experiments of Rosenow (8) seem to show that the streptococcus strains, which acquire an elective affinity for the gall-bladder, have also an affinity for muscular tissue, especially the myocardium. This confirms the clinical observation of the occurrence of cardiac muscle disease with cholecystitis. Therefore, surgery is indicated in appendicitis and cholecystitis to relieve the individual of a local menace to life, of reflex dyspepsia and quite as important to remove etiologic factors of systemic disease.

The morbid conditions of the rectum, which makes it a dangerous source of lymphogenous and hematogenous infection especially of colon bacilli and streptococci, should receive rational surgical treatment.

The focal acute and chronic infectious diseases of the pelvic organs of woman, particularly of the uterus in the puerperium and of the parametrium and fallopian tubes, are so important that they should be rationally managed and surgically treated when necessary to safeguard health and life.

The alleged etiological relation of chronic streptococcus infection to cystic degeneration of the ovary needs confirmatory bacteriologic research. This is especially needed if the supposed infectious cause of diseases of the ovary is accepted as an additional excuse for the too frequent sacrifice of the ovary for the numerous real and fancied ills of women.

The infectious foci of the male pelvic organs requires a management and surgical treatment which will remove a constant source of systemic diseases and in gonorrheal infection in addition, a source of the most frequent cause of pelvic disease of women, many of whom are morally innocent wives. As demonstrated by Sugimura (4) and Franke (5), lymphogenous infection in addition to other sources of hematogenous infection of the ureter, kidney pelvis and kidney, from the bladder, indicates additional reasons for effective treatment medical or surgical to overcome acute and chronic cystitis. So, too, may rational medical or surgical treatment of pyogenic and tuberculous kidney and kidney pelvis infections prevent corresponding infection of the ureter, bladder, other pelvic organs, and from all of these sources a general systemic infection.

Infected wounds, often insignificant, of the skin and mucous membranes and furuncles and purulent infection about the finger and toe nails should receive the management which is indicated by the rare, yet often serious, systemic infections which they may cause.

TREATMENT OF RESULTING ACUTE AND CHRONIC SYSTEMIC DISEASES

In the treatment of disease it is an axiom to remove the cause if possible. This law of good medical practice is applicable in diseases due to focal infection. In some acute diseases it is impossible to remove the focal disease, either because it is inaccessible or the serious con-

dition of the patient contraindicates it. In bacteriemia
due to puerperal sepsis, or to an infectious thrombophlebitis of the deep veins, surgery cannot be utilized
without danger of death from shock or from an over-
whelming degree of bacteriemia by a physical disturbance of the infected thrombus or other tissue sources of
the infection.

In acute rheumatic fever associated with endocarditis, pericarditis or a pancarditis, the serious
condition of the patient usually contraindicates tonsillectomy for the removal of the most general etiologic
focus. Experience teaches that removal of the tonsils
during an attack of acute rheumatic fever usually does
not modify the clinical course. It is the better practice
to remove the focal cause, wherever it may be, in the late
convalescence.

In mild rheumatic fever and in chronic infectious
forms of arthritis the focal cause should be removed
early. Even in these mild and chronic types of infectious arthritis and myositis one occasionally witnesses
serious results. A girl of eighteen who had suffered for
a year from a disabling chronic polyarthritis and myositis, due apparently to multiple chronic alveolar abscesses, had many teeth extracted and the alveolar abscesses curetted. Streptococcus bacteriemia developed
with acute hemorrhagic myositis, pleuritis, pericarditis,
myocarditis with submucous and subcutaneous hemorrhages and death. The streptococci isolated from the alveolar pus, the blood and after death from the muscles,
when injected intravenously into animals caused rheumatic arthritis, myositis, endocarditis and pericarditis.

A girl of ten, now a patient in the Presbyterian Hospital, suffered from a mild arthritis and myositis. The family physician had the enlarged and apparently infected tonsils removed. Immediately, there developed an acute general myositis, which gradually changed to a non-febrile type with much deformity due to the shortening of the muscles. Experience of this kind affords proof of the focal origin of certain systemic conditions and that the operative technic of removal of foci of infections should be of a kind which will not overwhelmingly inoculate the patient. In acute rheumatic infections the removal of the original focus, usually tonsillitis, may not prevent future attacks, for the streptococcus rheumaticus may occur in other focal sites, notably in alveolar abscess and maxillary sinusitis. The prompt removal of every recognizable local infection of the head, in people who suffer from repeated attacks of acute rheumatism, may prevent the disease. This result experience of recent years has conclusively proved. What has been said of the treatment of the acute rheumatic infections is also true of chorea. But experience has shown that arsenic does modify the course of chorea. It is interesting to note, in this connection, that arsenic has also a striking influence on the clinical course of rheumatic pericarditis and pleuritis. I have used cacodylate of soda as a relatively non-toxic form of arsenic in the treatment of chorea and of serofibrinous rheumatic pericarditis and pleuritis. From five to fifteen grains in divided doses, each twenty-four hours, injected deep in the muscles, has a remarkable effect within two or three days. The uniformly constant result suggests a chemotherapeutic result similar to that of salvarsan for spirochetes.

Salicylic acid seems to have a specific bactericidal effect upon the streptococcus rheumaticus if it is given in sufficient quantity in the first days. Large sterilizing doses given early seem necessary. Perhaps the streptococcus becomes immune to ineffectual doses of the drug, and this may explain the lack of specific effect in the prolonged clinical course. It is of interest to record the apparent good effect of large doses of salicylic acid during the first hours of acute appendicitis, which as we have noted may be caused by a modified strain of the streptococcus rheumaticus.

Acute gonorrheal arthritis must first be recognized by the pathognomonic signs sometimes present, purulent exudate in joints and tendon sheaths, the gonococcus in exudates and blood and the recognition of a focus in the genito-urinary tract. The specific von Pirquet skin and the complement fixation tests are not always to be relied upon in diagnosis unless suitably controlled, according to Irons (36), Irons and Nicoll (37). The almost uniform benefit of the early removal of the focal cause is notable in systemic gonococcus infection. Even with gonococcemia, if no involvement of the endocardium occurs and if there is no gonococcus thrombophlebitis, the removal of the focus is often followed by recovery. Purulent exudates must be surgically treated.

Malignant endocarditis of all types is usually fatal because the invading bacteria find lodgment and suitable conditions for growth and multiplication in large vegetations filled with thrombi or in the necrotic tissue of the valves and heart walls of the ulcerative form. This insures continued infection and increasing diminished resistance of the patient. Multiple embolism and the result upon all the involved organs hastens the fatal end. Drug treatment is unavailing.

Infectious acute nephritis due to the specific elective tissue affinity of certain bacteria, especially members of the streptococcus group, demands an early removal of the focal cause. By this means death may be prevented and if the anatomical injury of the kidney is not too great the function may be preserved to a degree consistent with health for many years. A woman of thirty years under treatment for chronic arthritis at the Presbyterian Hospital acquired coryza and an acute frontal sinusitis. Hemorrhagic nephritis immediately occurred, associated with some edema of the face, legs and dependent portions of the body. Drainage of the infected sinus was followed by rapid general improvement and a gradual disappearance of the albuminuria and the abnormal formed elements of the urine. One month later the urine and functional tests for phthalein, nitrogen and chlorid output were normal. A strain of streptococci, which was hemolytic, isolated from the exudate of the sinus, when injected intravenously into rabbits caused hemorrhagic nephritis.

Many like examples of improvement or recovery from acute hemorrhagic nephritis could be reported from our observation and the experience of others recorded in medical literature. So, too, one may cite examples of nephritis which have progressed to a hopeless stage due to repeated anatomical insults of the kidney by infectious microörganisms from the neglected focus.

Even types of chronic nephritis evidenced by albuminuria, cylindruria and more or less hyperarterial tension show manifest improvement by the removal of chronic focal infection of the dental alveoli, tonsils, sinuses, gall-bladder, appendix and pelvic organs. A rational after-treatment consisting of a properly selected diet and attention to personal hygiene is of course an important factor in the improved condition of these patients.

Appendicitis, acute and chronic, requires surgical intervention to conserve life and to obliterate a focal infection which may seriously infect other tissues through the lymph channel or blood stream. The incidence of appendicitis may be reduced by the prevention of focal infection about the head and by the early removal of existing foci.

Acute and chronic cholecystitis demand early surgical treatment to relieve pain and dyspepsia and quite as much to remove a dangerous focus of systemic infection, especially of the myocardium. Babcock (40) and others have noted the improvement of clinical chronic myocarditis by the drainage of a coexisting chronic cholecystitis. The prevention of focal infection of dental alveoli, tonsils and sinuses and the early removal of existing infection at these sites may diminish the incidence of cholecystitis and of gall-stones.

In the treatment of gastric and duodenal ulcer the experiments of Rosenow demand the primary removal of the etiologic foci of infection as a means of prevention of the recurrence of the ulcer through reinfection. A coincident rational medical management if consistently carried out, as advised by Sippy (56), may be successful in healing the ulcer. Surgical treatment is indicated when the unhealed ulcer or the scar produces deformities which persistently interfere with gastric and intestinal function and also when accidents, like perforation and medically unmanageable hemorrhage, occur.

Recurring erythema nodosum alone or as a part of the syndrome described by Osler (17) may be entirely controlled by the removal of the etiologic infectious focus. A young woman of twenty-four years had recurring attacks of erythematous nodes of the arms and lower extremities, associated with mild arthritis. She suffered from a chronic maxillary sinusitis. Drainage of the sinus gave coincident freedom from the nodes and arthritis. After three months a recurrence of the systemic disease proved to be due to a corresponding recurrence of the sinus infection. Complete obliteration of the sinus infection has been followed by the continued absence of the attacks of arthritis and erythematous nodes for three years.

A young married woman of twenty-six had recurrent attacks of erythematous nodes and muscular soreness for a year. She had also frequent mild tonsillitis and pharyngitis. Enucleation of the tonsils was followed by the absence of erythematous nodes for nearly a year, then a recurrence. Re-examination revealed the presence of an infected lower pole of one tonsil. The removal of the remaining portion of infected tonsil has resulted in the permanent cessation of the systemic disease.

The relation of focal infection to acute pancreatitis often associated with cholecystitis has been noted. Early surgical intervention to relieve the acute process is imperatively demanded. Chronic pancreatitis is of especial interest because of the relation the internal secretion of the gland bears to carbohydrate metabolism. The probable infectious origin of chronic pancreatitis as well as the acute process from streptococcus foci, affords an interesting problem for clinical investigation in the management of diabetes mellitus. We have removed existing focal infection about the head of diabetic patients, have inoculated animals with the isolated streptococcus strains, and have kept the patients under clinical observation. The results have not been uniform enough to warrant a conclusive statement at this time.

Chronic pancreatitis which is etiologically related to chronic cholecystitis and calculous cholecystitis as determined by Opie (32) may disappear clinically by the surgical removal of the etiologic factors.

Osteomyelitis may not be benefited by the removal of the pyogenic bacteria containing focus of the tonsils, jaws, sinuses and other tissues. Rationally the etiologic focus should be removed coincidentally with the surgical treatment of the bone infection.

Infectious thyroiditis which occurs during a general infection, like rheumatic fever, may subside during convalescence from the general infection. When infectious goiter is due to a focal infection of the tonsils and alveolar abscess, removal of the focus is usually followed by diminution in the size of the gland and by a disappearance of the symptoms of thyroid intoxication. This has been demonstrated in many individuals, chiefly young women patients. The majority of these women were overworked and often poorly nourished, with resulting lowered immunity to the focal infection. Many of the patients are under continued observation and without exception there has been no instance of relapse of the goiter or of hyperthyroidism.

Hematogenous focal infection of the nervous apparatus, involving the gasserian and posterior spinal root ganglia and spinal cord, affords confirmation of the infectious nature of herpes, of insular sclerosis and myelitis of the spinal cord. Removal of the primary etiologic foci of infection about the upper air tract and mouth may modify favorably the course of the spinal cord infection.

The treatment of chronic types of infectious arthritis and myositis is usually neglected or so irrationally conducted that failure to benefit the sufferer is the usual result. This unfortunate condition is due chiefly to a want of knowledge by most physicians of the principal factors which cause the morbid tissue changes. An attempt was made to explain these principles in Lecture IV.

In the treatment the primary necessity is to obtain a knowledge of the patient's general condition and to locate existing foci of infection which may have been the chief primary cause, or still continue to be sources of systemic infection. The result of rational management will depend, partly in any event, upon the degree and character of the morbid tissue changes in the joints and muscles, upon the command one may have in the management and upon the age of the patient. Destructive lesions of bones and cartilege, bony ankylosis, extensive sclerotic changes and atrophy of muscles cannot be repaired. Indeed because of the destruction of blood vessels and the resulting want of nutrition, continued retrograde metabolism favors the change of the connective tissue group, tendons, aponeurosis, ligament and cartilage into bone. This is true of all types of chronic infectious non-purulent arthritis of whatever bacterial type. Therefore, if the treatment is to result in the arrest of the disease with advanced morbid anatomical changes or in the recovery of those with non-destructive morbid tissue changes, institutional care is required to insure the necessary command of the patient over a sufficiently long period of time to remove all focal sources of infection, to build up general nutrition and to restore as nearly as possible the blood circulation in the infected tissues. This method of management is necessary to stop the sources of systemic infection, to build up the body defenses against the existing systemic infection and to improve the general and local nutrition as the chief means of arresting retrograde metabolism and at the same time to promote resolution of the morbid infectious processes. Rationally the younger the patient the readier will be the response to the management.

In the preliminary general examination one may need the aid of qualified specialists in the examination of the nasopharynx, ears, accessory sinuses, pelvic organs and

blood, and Röntgen films of jaws and plates of joints
to locate etiologic infectious foci and to determine the
degree of the joint changes. Microscopic examination
and cultures of blood, accessible exudates of joints and
of foci in the head, pelvis and elsewhere and of the urine
and feces may give valuable information of the character of the bacterial infection. Intravenous injection
of the nascent cultures of the bacteria into animals may
produce lesions corresponding with the morbid changes
of the patients' tissues. With the consent of the patient
always, a harmless and, under local anesthesia, painless
removal of pieces of infected muscle, joint capsule,
fibrous nodes and lymph nodes proximal to the infected
tissues enables one to study the morbid histology and
with a proper technic to isolate the causative infectious
microörganisms from the tissues. But important as the
study of the exudates, tissues and bacteria may be, the
real and important principle is to know all that one
may of the physical condition of the patient. Following this diagnosis the management includes:

1.   The removal of all primary and, if necessary, all
secondary foci of infection.   To make sure that all
sources of focal infection have been obliterated, repeated
examination should be made. Buried tonsillar tissue
may be left at the primary tonsillectomy. An infected
sinus may not have been adequately treated. Alveolar
abscess may finally require the extraction of the tooth.
An apparently cured gonococcus infection of the prostate and seminal vesicles may recur. Constant vigilance
is necessary to insure the abolition of continued systemic
reinfection.

2. To build up the natural defenses of the body. To accomplish this involves close attention to important principles including mental and physical rest, nourishing food, restorative tonics when indicated, cheerful environment, good air and sunshine and with some patients the use of suitable bacterial antigens as vaccines to stimulate the formation of specific antibodies in the tissues of the patient. Mental and physical rest must be rationally supervised to meet the idiosyncrasies of the individual. Isolation and continuous bed confinement may be exchanged for open ward and partial chair treatment to meet the viewpoint of the patient and thus promote the most efficient rest of mind and body. This absolute rest must be maintained until in febrile cases all fever shall have disappeared and also until the severe soreness of the joints and muscles aggravated by motion shall have diminished, for until then the exercise of infected tissues lowers the natural resistance to infection and thereby increases the infection of the joints and muscles. Often the temporary application of restraining bandages, splints and casts may favor the diminution of the local infection. The usually poor general nutrition of patients with chronic infectious arthritis calls for a generous mixed diet including an abundance of fats, oils, green vegetables and fruits. The emaciated tissues demand a full allowance of protein-containing food, both animal and vegetable. A plentiful amount of water, milk, buttermilk, cream and fruit juices must be taken.

When necessary, hematinic and other tonics, laxatives, and simple analgesic palliatives, such as the salicylic acid compounds, may be judiciously given. There are no specific drugs to be used and narcotics should be avoided in these chronic diseases.

The mental depression of this class of patients retards improvement, hence the need of a constant, cheerful environment and an optimistic attitude of all who come in contact with them.

With the sources of systemic infection obliterated, and the existing systemic infection diminished or entirely controlled by the management described, other measures must be added to the treatment which may stop further retrograde metabolism, and in favorable conditions may result in the restoration of normal anatomical and functional conditions of the tissues of the joints and muscles.

These measures are so important that the failure to apply them adequately means failure in the whole management. The object of their use is to attempt to restore nutrition to the starved tissues of joints and muscles which have been deprived more or less of blood and oxygen by the embolic mode of repeated infection from the primary focus, for as long as the infected tissues are starved, conditions exist which are favorable to continued infection and furthermore, local malnutrition leads to retrograde tissue metabolism.

In addition to the measures already advised to increase the general nutrition, the local malnutrition may be wholly or partly overcome by an improvement of the general and local blood circulation. The measures consist of hydrotherapy, active and passive exercise, local application of superheated dry air and the Bier blood congestion method by the application of the rubber bandage.

Hydrotherapy in the form of alternating hot and cold shower or spray baths, applied daily for a few minutes, flushes the blood to all the parts of the body without fatigue to the patient. If the force with which the water strikes the body is relatively high, the improvement of the circulation is greater. The tonic effect upon the circulatory organs of the application of cold water to the skin is well known. A cold plunge bath is disagreeable to these enervated patients. The alternating hot-cold spray repeated several times in a few minutes, is borne without complaint, and the result is quite as good as the use of the cold bath alone. In the absence of facilities for applying shower or spray baths, salt glows and alcohol rubs may be utilized as poor substitutes of the cold bath.

Passive exercise of joints and muscles may be given by nurses or more efficiently by individuals trained to give massage. Mechanical aids in the form of the Zander apparatus if rationally used give good results.

Active calisthenic exercises may be so taught that under proper supervision each patient will have the benefit of periods of exercise modified to meet individual conditions.

Other active exercise, like walking, riding, driving, swimming and gymnastic work, may be taken up at the proper time. An individual qualified by education and experience should have the supervision of the treatment by baths, and mechanotherapy. Every general hospital should have a mechanotherapeutic department with a qualified director for the treatment at the right stage of the management of the large number of patients, in all communities, who suffer from chronic infectious arthritis and of other chronic diseases. If rationally and efficiently managed many would be restored to health, while in others with more advanced morbid anatomical changes the further progress of disease would be more or less checked and an improvement of function would be gained.

SERUM AND VACCINE THERAPY

Serum Therapy

The prophylactic and therapeutic use of antitoxic sera in diphtheria and tetanus is established upon a scientific basis. The specific neutralization of the poison excreted by the exotoxic bacillus of diphtheria and bacillus of tetanus, when the respective antitoxic serum is properly administered, may be accurately ascertained by clinical and laboratory methods.

The use of specific antisera in the treatment of diseases caused by endotoxic bacteria has been far from successful. The principle upon which the value of antisera is based, is that when injected subcutaneously, there will be aroused in the body of the patient specific defensive forces, in the form of antibodies, leukocytic phagocytosis and bactericidal substances which may favorably modify the course of the disease. In epidemic cerebrospinal meningitis the specific antimeningococcal serum of Flexner, when injected directly into the spinal subarachnoid space, apparently has specific bactericidal properties. The injected serum probably arouses tissue reactions, which mobilizes the defenses of the body, increasing cellular phagocytosis, digestion of the invading meningococci and even acting directly as a bactericide. Other therapeutic antisera obtained by immunizing animals with strains of the streptococcus, pneumococcus, bacillus of dysentery and other endotoxic bacteria have not given uniform results. The failure of these sera generally now is recognized to be due to several factors, including the existence of variant strains of bacteria which may not be differentiated morphologically. Moreover, there may be a marked difference in the various strains in pathogenicity and virulence and in the tissue reactions of the infected individual. Each strain may arouse specific effects and the results thereof will be influenced only by the therapeutic serum obtained from an animal immunized with a like strain. This principle has been successfully utilized by Cole and his co-workers in pneumonia. They have classified the pneumococcus into four types, of which types I, II and III represent single specific strains and type IV a group of strains unlike the first three types. The antiserum must be prepared by immunizing an animal with the type of pneumococcus which is to be attacked. The same principle has been proved to exist in reference to the pathogenic strains of streptococci and of the strains of the bacillus of dysentery. The principle of the necessary possession of "type" specificity of the bacteria used in the production of antisera to obtain anything like satisfactory therapeutic results has been apparently established. While it may not prove to be a principle to be applied to the preparation of antisera of all endotoxic, pathogenic bacteria, perhaps to a few only, yet there is in its adoption the hope that a broader field of specific antiserum treatment may be developed.

In our study of focal and systemic infections we used the antiserum of the horse immunized with strains of streptococcus viridans in the treatment of streptococcus viridans endocarditis and in chronic arthritis without notable good effect. Apparently unavoidable anaphylactic shock and other objectionable effects compelled us to abandon its use. Therefore, the production of and the use of antisera in the treatment of diseases due to focal infection present problems which present knowledge may not solve.

Vaccine Therapy

We know that a degree of immunity to some infectious diseases may be produced in man and animals by inoculation with non-lethal doses of living or dead pathogenic bacteria. In a few diseases, a mild form of infection or intoxication is produced by the inoculation with resulting immunity of variable duration. Attenuation of the virulence of living virus used for inoculation has been successfully practiced to produce a mild disease which affords protection to the protean malady. Vaccinia in man produced by inoculation with cowpox protects against variola. Inoculation with living or dead typhoid bacteria and paratyphoid bacilli with proper technic will afford immunity of variable time duration to typhoid and paratyphoid fevers. These examples of the use of vaccines in *prophylaxis* have a very limited application in practice. Probably the field of application may become broader when we finally recognize the specific etiologic microörganisms of all infectious diseases which usually give a lasting immunity by one attack. Then, as in typhoid fever, prophylactic vaccination may become of the greatest use in preventive medicine.

Vaccination with attenuated virus during a long inoculation stage of infection, as successfully practiced by Pasteur in man bitten by animals suffering with rabies, will probably not be applicable in other infections which have comparatively shorter incubation stages. The present use of *therapeutic* vaccines is based upon less stable scientific principles. In 1902 Wright evolved the use of autogenous vaccines in chronic infectious diseases. He believed that the natural defenses of the body, exhausted by long infection, would be increased and mobilized by inoculation with microörganisms of the same type and kind which caused the chronic disease. He judged the improvement in the defensive forces of the patient's body after autogenous vaccination by estimating the opsonins in the patient's blood. He argued that with an increase of specific antibodies in the blood of the patient, the fibrinoplastic exudative barrier surrounding local infectious processes, which afforded protection to the localized bacteria, would be broken down by the mobilization of immune substances. The bacteria so exposed would then be readily overcome. Thus furunculosis of the skin, due usually to a staphylococcus, was more readily overcome by autogenous staphylococcus vaccine.

It would seem rational, too, that a general chronic

infectious process would be more readily overcome by
the use of an autogenous vaccine which would increase
the natural defenses of the body which have become exhausted by the long battle with the invading bacteria.
Unfortunately the question involves many unknown factors. A certain type of pathogenic bacterium, used as
an antigen, may excite the formation of antibodies in
the nature of opsonins, agglutinins, precipitins, leukocytosis, phagocytosis and other offensive or defensive processes, but we may not depend upon a similar result with
other pathogenic bacteria etiologically related to other
infectious diseases. We cannot, from present knowledge, definitely expect the same tissue reactions and resulting formation of immune substances in man and
laboratory animals infected with the same type of infectious bacteria. Indeed the resulting tissue reactions
and formation of defensive and offensive substances to
a strain of pathogenic microörganisms may differ in degree and kind in human beings, dependent on age, race,
occupation and other factors. Variations of type of
strains of pathogenic bacteria with corresponding differences in the tissue reactions of infected individuals,
is an important factor in immunological experimentation. We know that the pneumococcus and strains of
streptococci not only differ in type, but also differ in
virulence, and that each type probably arouses defensive
and offensive forces in the infected individual, differing
more or less for each type; and possibly the tissue reactions are still further modified by the degree of virulence of the invading bacteria. Pathogenic bacteria may
possess a mono- or polytropism; that is, an elective affin-

ity for a certain kind of tissue or for several kinds of tissues. Therefore, if specific vaccine is necessary to arouse specific immune substances to combat offensively or defensively the invading infectious bacteria, it implies the use of an autogenous antigen. In this sense an autogenous vaccine means the use of dead bacteria, proved to be of the same specific type in virulence and tropism as that which causes the infection of the individual who receives the vaccine. In chronic infectious diseases, it is often difficult to isolate definitely the microörganisms which are the real etiologic factors in a given case. Without an accurate bacterial diagnosis one is unable to discuss the other vexatious problems which must be considered in the elaboration and use of the autogenous vaccine.

In our work we have isolated the suspected bacteria from the blood, lymph nodes, fibrous nodes, joint exudates, joint tissues, muscles, skin and other infected tissues of patients. To ascertain the tissue tropism we have injected animals intravenously and from the infected tissues of the experimental animals, have again isolated the bacteria. Vaccines have been prepared from cultures made from the microörganisms isolated from patients and also from the cultures derived from patients after animal passage with especial regard to tissue tropism. We have also sensitized some of these vaccines with antiserum.

We have used these autogenous vaccines in the treatment of many types of chronic infectious disease. More than five hundred patients suffering with infectious arthritis have received the vaccines subcutaneously in doses varying from 10,000,000 to 2,000,000,000 and more, given every five to seven days, and in rare instances daily. The focal, local and general reaction of patients was carefully noted. For two years the opsonic index and the phagocytic index of each patient were estimated painstakingly before and after each vaccination.

The difficulty of estimating the opsonins and the final conclusion that the opsonic index obtained by the most careful technic is unreliable led us to abandon that method of estimating the results of autogenous vaccination.

In place thereof we managed some patients with and some without vaccination, but all of them upon the same hygienic treatment. The final result was quite as satisfactory without as with vaccine, in patients suffering with chronic infectious arthritis and acute rheumatism.

Patients suffering with chronic streptococcus viridans endocarditis were not benefited by autogenous vaccines. Indeed I believe some of them were made distinctly worse when moderately large doses of vaccines were used.

The problems which confront the clinician in the use of therapeutic vaccines, must be solved by the immunologist. The views of Theobald Smith (39), Richard M. Pearce (38) and others in regard to therapeutic vaccines should be read by every clinician.

Based upon the work of Wright, but disregardful of the principles developed by him, therapeutic vaccination has progressed in this country into an irrational fad which is intensified and made degrading to the medical profession and harmful to the patients by commercial greed.

We are forgetful of the principles of medical practice of our fathers. They recognized the influence of old age, exposure to extreme cold, poverty and poor nutrition, physical and mental exhaustion, faulty personal hygiene and other debility-producing factors in the causation and also in the prolongation of infectious and other diseases. They also recognized the necessity of the removal as far as possible of all these contributory etiologic factors in the management of the patient. The modern vaccinationist pins his faith on the advertised specific virtues of stock vaccines, which he may employ in polyvalent form to insure a sure-shot effect. He believes vaccines will arouse specific defenses in the tissues of the patient in spite of all contributory etiologic factors of disease. Therefore, the rational diet, proper baths, passive and active exercise, correction of personal uncleanliness and alcohol misuse are neglected. The practitioner usually is ignorant of all laws of immunology. It is this want of knowledge which makes him believe the ridiculous statements made by the manufacturers of vaccines.

Modern experimental investigation of the physiologic action of drugs has done much to restrict the abuse of drug therapy of the past. So, too, must the practitioner be made acquainted with what we know and do not know of immunology. We must restrict the therapeutic use of bacterial antigens to those conditions which the known laws of immunity and scientific clinical experience have proved to be safe and of value.

The Therapeutic Use of Non-specific Protein Antigens Injected Intravenously

In recent time the intravenous injection of non-specific proteins (bacterial and others) has been used in the treatment of both acute and chronic infectious disease. The phenomena aroused by a proper intravenous dosage consist of a chill followed by high fever, great general discomfort, usually a relatively slow pulse rate, leukocytosis sometimes of a high degree, not infrequently preceded by an immediate leukopenia. Gay and Chickering (49) have used the protein, non-toxic remnant of the typhoid bacillus by intravenous injection in the treatment of typhoid fever. The characteristic phenomena noted above resulted. When used after the first week of typhoid fever, the reaction was followed by a critical fall of the temperature and convalesence was established in 41.5 per cent. A gradual fall of temperature occurred with abbreviation of the course in 24.5 per cent. and no permanent benefit occurred in 34 per cent. of the patients treated. We have used the non-toxic protein remnant of pneumococci obtained by autolysis of the bacteria, first suggested by E. C. Rosenow, in pneumonia. When injected intravenously, the typical phenomena occurred with apparent beneficial effect, which was most marked if used early in the course of the disease.

In acute rheumatism and also in chronic infectious arthritis, astonishing beneficial effects have been noted in a few instances from the intravenous injection of typhoid, of colon and of other non-specific protein antigens. Jobling and Peterson (48) injected animals intravenously with dead bacteria and found that non-specific ferments were mobilized. They believe that these ferments are bactericidal and that at the same time'toxic substances are rendered non-toxic. The suggestion has been made that the severe reaction caused by the intravenous injection of a foreign protein, is followed by a condition of refraction (anti-anaphylaxis) and the organism fails to react to the invading bacteria. Jobling believes that it will be possible in the near future to use intravenously the non-toxic portion of protein to excite the mobilization of the helpful ferments without the painful, disagreeable and even dangerous clinical phenomena which attend the intravenous use of unmodified protein antigen. The mode of action of the non-specific albumose antigens, injected intravenously, is not well understood. Their use in acute and chronic infectious diseases affords a fruitful field of combined research by the immunologist and clinician.

BIBLIOGRAPHY

1. BASS, C. C., and JOHNS, F. M. "Pyorrhea Dentalis and Alveolaris." *The Jour. A. M. A.*, 1915, LXIV, 553.

2. BARRETT, M. F. Preliminary Report, *Dental Cosmos*, 1914, LVI, 948.

3. SMITH, ALLEN J., MIDDLETON, W. S., and BARRETT, M. F. "Tonsils as a Habitat of Oral Endamebas," *The Jour. A. M. A.*, 1914, LXIII, 1746.

4. SUGIMURA, S. "Ueber die Beteilung der Ureteren an den akuten Blasen entzündengen nebst Bemerkungen über ihre Fortleitung durch die Lymphbahnen der Ureteren." *Virchow Arch.*, CCVI, 20.

5. FRANKE, CARL. "Die Koliinfection des Harnapparats und deren Therapie." *Ergabniss d. Chirurg. u. Orthopöd.*, 1913, VII, 671.

6. DICK, GEO. F., and DICK, GLADYS R. "The Bacteriology of the Urine in Non-suppurative Nephritis." *The Jour. A. M. A.*, 1915, LXV, 6.

7. KOLLE, W., and WASSERMANN, A. "Latency of Infectious Bacteria." *Hand Buch der Path. Mikroorganismen*, 1903, I, 147.

8. ROSENOW, E. C. "Immunological and Experimental Studies on Pneumococcus and Streptococcus Endocarditis" (Chronic Septic Endocarditis). *Jour. Inf. Dis.*, 1909, VI, 245.

——. "A Study of Pneumococci from Cases of Infectious Endocarditis." *Jour. Inf. Dis.*, 1910, VII, 411.

——. "Immunological Studies in Chronic Pneumococcus Endocarditis." *Jour. Inf. Dis.*, 1910, VII, 429.

——. "Transmutation Within the Streptococcus-Pneumococcus Group." *Jour. Inf. Dis.*, 1914, XIV, I.

Rosenow, E. C. "The Etiology of Acute Rheumatism, Articular and Muscular." *Jour. Inf. Dis.*, 1914, XIV, 61.

——. "The Bacteriology of Appendicitis and Its Production by Intravenous Injection of Streptococci and Colon Bacilli." *Jour. Inf. Dis.*, 1915, XVI, 240.

——. "The Etiology and Experimental Production of Erythema Nodosum." *Jour. Inf. Dis.*, 1915, XVI, 367.

8. Rosenow, E. C., and Sanford, A. H. "The Bacteriology of Ulcer of the Stomach and Duodenum in Man." *Jour. Inf. Dis.*, 1915, XVII, 219.

8. Rosenow, E. C. "The Newer Bacteriology of Various Infections as Determined by Special Methods." *The Jour. A. M. A.*, 1914, LXIII, 903.

——. "Bacteriology of Cholecystitis and Its Production by Injection of Streptococci." *The Jour. A. M. A.*, 1914, LXIII, 1835.

8. Rosenow, E. C., and Ofterdal, Sverri. "The Etiology and Experimental Production of Herpes Zoster." *The Jour. A. M. A.*, 1915, LXIV, 1968.

8. Rosenow, E. C. "Iritis and Other Ocular Lesions on Intravenous Injection of Streptococci." *Jour. Inf. Dis.*, 1915, XVII, 403.

9. Billings, Frank. "Chronic Focal Infections and Their Etiologic Relations to Arthritis and Nephritis." *Arch. Int. Med.*, 1912, IX, 484.

——. "Chronic Focal Infections as a Causative Factor in Chronic Arthritis." *The Jour. A. M. A.*, 1913, LXI, 819.

——. "Chronic Infectious Endocarditis." *The Arch. Int. Med.*, 1909, IV, 409.

——. "Clinical Aspect and Medical Management of Arthritis Deformans." *Ill. Med. Jour.*, 1914, XXV, 11.

——. "Focal Infection: Its Broader Application in the Etiology of General Disease." *The Jour. A. M. A.*, 1914, LXIII, 899.

Billings, Frank. "Systemic Diseases of Focal Origin." *Forchheimer's Therapeusis*, 1914, V, 169.

10. Schottmüller, H. "Die Artuntersuchendung der für Menschen Pathogenen Streptokokken durch Blutagar." *Münch. Med. Wchnschr.*, 1903, L, 849.

———. "Zür Aetiologie der Pneumonie Cruposa." *Münch. Med. Wchnschr.*, 1905, LII, 30.

———. "Endocarditis Lenta." *Münch. Klin. Wchnschr.*, 1910, 880 (quoted by Libman).

11. Cole, Rufus, and Dochez, A. R. "Report of Studies in Pneumonia." *Trans. Assn. Am. Phys.*, 1913, XXVIII, 606.

12. Haessli, Hans. "Der Verhalten der Streptokokken Gegenüber Plasma und Serum und ihre Umzüchtung." *Mitth. a. d. Hamb. Staats Krankenamst*, 1910, XL, 10.

13. Forssner, G. "Renale Lokalisation nach intravenösen Injektionen mit einer dem Nierengewebe experimental angepassten Streptokokken cultur." *Nord. Med. Arkiv.*, 1902, XXXV, 1-56.

14. Poynton, F. J., and Paine, A. "The Etiology of Rheumatic Fever." *The Lancet*, 1900, II, 861.

———. "A Further Contribution to the Study of Rheumatism; the Experimental Production of Appendicitis by the Intravenous Inoculation of the Diplococcus." *The Lancet*, 1911, II.

———. "Observations Upon the Arthritis Produced in Rabbits by the Intravenous Inoculation of a Diplococcus Isolated from Cases of Rheumatism." *Trans. Path. Soc.*, London, 1904.

———. "Observations Upon Certain Forms of Arthritis." *Br. Med. Jour.*, 1902, II, 1414.

———. "The Pathogenesis of Rheumatic Fever." *Trans. Path. Soc.*, London, 1901.

———. "The Relation of Malignant to Rheumatic Endocarditis." *The Lancet*, 1902, I, 1036.

Poynton, F. J., and Paine, A. "Remarks on the Infectious Nature of Rheumatic Fever, Illustrated by the Study of a Fatal Case." *Br. Med. Jour.*, 1904, I.

———. "Some Further Investigations and Observations Upon the Pathology of Rheumatic Fever." *The Lancet*, 1910, I, 1524.

15. Beattie, James. "Acute Rheumatism." *Edinb. Med. Jour.*, 1904.

16. Walker, E. W. A., and Ryffel, J. H. "The Pathology of Acute Rheumatism and Allied Disorders." *Br. Med. Jour.*, 1903, II, 659.

17. Osler, Wm. "Chronic Infectious Endocarditis." *Quar. Jour. Med.*, 1909, II, 219.

———. "On the Visceral Complications of Erythema Exudativum Multiforme." *Am. Jour. Med. Sci.*, 1895, CX, 629.

18. Horder, Thomas J. "Infective Endocarditis." *Quar. Jour. Med.*, 1909, II, 289.

19. Libman, E., and Celler, H. L. "The Etiology of Subacute Infective Endocarditis." *Jour. Am. Med. Sci.*, 1910, CXL, 516.

20. Libman, E. "A Study of the Lesions of Subacute Bacterial Endocarditis with Peculiar Reference to Healing or Healed Lesions, with Clinical Notes." *Jour. Am. Med. Sci.*, 1912, CXLIV, 313.

21. Herrick, James B. "The Healing of Ulcerative Endocarditis." *Med. News*, 1902, XXXI, 10.

22. Lenhartz, H. "Ueber die Septische Endocarditis." *Münch. Med. Wchschr.*, 1901, XLVIII, 28.

23. Baehr, Geo. "Glomerular Lesions of Subacute Bacterial Endocarditis." *Jour. Am. Med. Sci.*, 1912, CXLIV, 327.

24. Lohlein, M. "Ueber hämorrhagische Nieren Affektionen bei Chronischer Ulcerösen Endokarditis." *Med. Klin.*, 1910, VI, 10.

25. KRETZ, RICHARD. "Angina und Septische Infektion."
    Zeitschr. f. Heilkund., 1907, XXVIII, 296.

26. CANNON, DR. "Ueber die Frage der hämatogenen In-
    fektion bei Appendicitis und Cholecystitis." *Deutsch.
    Zeitschr. f. Chir.*, 1908, XCV, 21.

27. GHON, A., and NAMBA, K. "Zur Frage über die Genese
    der Appendicitis." *Beitrag. z. Path. Anat. u. z.
    Algem. Path.*, 1912, LII, 130.

28. ADRIAN, C. "Die Appendicitis als Folge einer Allgemei-
    nerkrankung." Klinisches und Experimentelles. *Mit-
    teil, a. d. Grenzgeb. d. Med. u. Chir.*, 1901, VII,
    407.

29. HEYDE, M. "Bakteriologische und Experimentelle
    Untersuchungen zur Aetologie der Wurmfort-
    sätzentzüngen (mitt besondere Berücksichtigung der
    Anaëroben Bakterien)." *Beitr. z. Klin. Chir.*, 1911,
    LXXVI, I.

30. ASCHOFF, L. "Pathogenese und Ätiologie der Appen-
    dicitis." *Ergebnisse d. Inner Med. u. Kinderheil-
    kund*, 1912, IX, 1.

31. VINCENT, H. "Sur la thyroidism dans la rheumatisme
    aigu, et sur l'origine rheumatismale de certain cas
    du goitre exophthalmique." *Compt. rend. Soc. de
    Biol.*, 1907, LXIII, 389.

——. "Rapports de la maladie Basedow avec la rheumatisme
    aigu." *Bull. de la Soc. Med. de Paris*, 1907, XXIV,
    1286; *Semaine Med.*, 1907, Mar. 20, 143, *Ibid.*, 1907,
    Nov. 21, 575; *Ibid.*, 1908, Jan. 1, 47; *Ibid.*, 1908,
    Oct. 28, 527.

32. OPIE, E. L. "The Etiology of Acute Hemorrhagic
    Pancreatitis." *J. H. H. Bull.*, 1901, 182.

33. DAVIS, D. J. "Bacteriological and Experimental Ob-
    servations on Focal Infection." *Arch. Int. Med.*,
    1912, 505.

34. JACKSON, LELIA. "Experimental Rheumatic Myocar-
    ditis." *Jour. Inf. Dis.*, 1912, XI, 240.

35. LE COUNT, E. R., and JACKSON, LELIA. "The Renal Changes in Rabbits Inoculated with Streptococci." *Jour. Inf. Dis.*, 1914, XV, 389.

36. IRONS, ERNEST E. "Bacteriology and Immunity. Studies in Gonococcal Immunity." *Trans. XVIIth Internat. Med. Cong.*, 1913, 87.

37. IRONS, ERNEST E., and NICOLL, H. K. "Complement Fixation in the Diagnosis of Gonococcal Infections." *Jour. Inf. Dis.*, 1915, XVI, 303.

38. PEARCE, RICHARD M. "The Scientific Basis of Vaccine Therapy." *The Jour. A. M. A.*, 1913, LXI, 2115.

39. SMITH, THEOBALD. "An Attempt to Interpret Present-Day Uses of Vaccine." *The Jour. A. M. A.*, 1913, LX, 1591.

——. "Theobald Smith Phenomena" (Anaphylaxis). Referred to by many experimental workers. See *Jour. A. M. A.*, 1906, 1910, and Lewis, P. A., *Jour. Exper. Med.*, 1908, X, 1.

40. BABCOCK, ROBT. H. "Chronic Cholecystitis as a Cause of Myocardial Incompetence." *Jour. A. M. A.*, 1909, LII, 1904.

41. NICHOLS, EDWARD H., and RICHARDSON, FRANK L. "Arthritis Deformans." *Jour. Med. Research*, 1909; N. S., XVI, 149.

42. WEIL, RICHARD. "Anaphylaxis and Its Relation to Problems of Human Disease." *Cinn. Lancet Clinic*, 1913, Nov. 19.

——. "Studies in Anaphylaxis. Desensitization; Its Theoretical and Practical Significance." *The Jour. of Med. Research*, 1913, New Series, XXIV, 233.

——. "Studies in Anaphylaxis." *The Jour. Med. Research*, 1914, New Series, XXV, 299.

43. VON PIRQUET, C. E. "Allergy." *Arch. Int. Med.*, 1911, VII, 259.

44. ROSENAU, M. L., and ANDERSON, JOHN F. "Hypersusceptibility." *Jour. A. M. A.*, 1906, XLVII, 1007.

ROSENAU, M. L., and ANDERSON, JOHN F. "A Study of the Cause of Sudden Death, Following the Injection of Horse Serum." 1906, *Hygienic Laboratory Bul.*, No. 29.

——. "Studies on Hypersusceptibility and Immunity." 1907, *Hygienic Laboratory Bul.*, No. 36.

——. "Further Studies Upon the Phenomenon of Anaphylaxis." 1909, *Hygienic Laboratory Bul.*, No. 50.

45. VAUGHAN, V. C. "Protein Split Products in Relation to Immunity and Disease." Lea & Febiger, Philadelphia, 1913.

46. AUER, J., and LEWIS, PAUL L. "Acute Anaphylactic Death in Guinea Pigs." *Jour. A. M. A.*, 1909, LIII, 458, and *Jour. Exper. Med.*, 1910, XII, 151.

47. PARK, W. H. "A Critical Study of the Results of Serum Therapy in the Diseases of Man." *The Harvey Lectures*, 1905-6, 101, Lippincott.

48. JOBLING, JAMES W., and PETERSEN. "Bacterio Therapy in Typhoid Fever." *Jour. A. M. A.*, 1915, LXV, 515.

49. GAY, FREDERICK P., and CHICKERING, HENRY T. "Treatment of Typhoid Fever by Intravenous Injections of Polyvalent Sensitized Typhoid Vaccine Sediment." *The Arch. of Int. Med.*, 1916, XVII, 303.

50. HASTINGS, T. W. "Complement Fixation Tests in Chronic Infective Deforming Arthritis and Arthritis Deformans." *Jour. Exper. Med.*, 1914, XX, 52.

——. "Concerning a Polyvalent Antigen for the Complement Fixation Test for Streptococcus Viridans Infection." *Jour. Exper. Med.*, 1914, XX, 72.

51. PHILLIPS, LLEWELLYN. "Emetine in Amebiasis." *Jour. Trop. Med. and Hygiene*, 1914, Aug. 15.

52. MELTZER, S. J. "Bronchial Asthma as a Phenomenon of Anaphylaxis." *Jour. A. M. A.*, 1910, LV, 1021.

53. JOBLING, J. W., PETERSEN, W. F., and EGGSTEIN, A. A. "The Mechanism of Anaphylactic Shock. Studies

on Ferment Action." *Jour. Exper. Med.*, 1914, XX, 401, and 1915, XXII, 401.

54. KLOTZ, OSKAR. "Experimental Bacterial Interstitial Nephritis." *Trans. Assoc. American Physicians*, 1914, XXIX, 49.

55. OPHULS, W. "Subacute and Chronic Nephritis as Found In One Thousand Unselected Autopsies." *Arch. Int. Med.*, 1912, IX, 156.

56. SIPPY, B. W. "Gastric and Duodenal Ulcer, Medical Care by an Efficient Removal of Gastric Juice Corrosion." *Jour. A. M. A.*, 1915, LXIV, 1628.

57. THAYER, W. S. "On Gonorrheal Septicemia and Endocarditis." *Amer. Jour. Med. Sci.*, Nov., 1905, new series, CXXXI, 751.

www.ingramcontent.com/pod-product-compliance
Lightning Source LLC
Chambersburg PA
CBHW030444290526
45786CB00001B/435